An Apocryphal Dictionary of Psychoanalysis

An Apocryphal Dictionary of Psychoanalysis is a book of transpositions, collecting together the author's clinical vignettes, enigmatic objects, stray thoughts, projects, images, notes from readings, and musings; but also remarks on films and exhibitions, memories, episodes from daily life, summaries of papers to write, questions, doubts and obsessions – all of which have shaped the author's understanding of psychoanalysis.

Born from moments in which the author has sensed a solution for problems encountered in daily work or for obscure but exciting points of the theory, the entries are ordered in an apocryphal manner, offering a personal and challenging view of psychoanalysis. Like small epiphanies in which there is always an emotion – be it that of amusement, astonishment, gratitude, sadness, joy – they express the style of the analyst and of the person in treating mental suffering and give a glimpse into the imaginary which nurtures it. Ideas for psychoanalysis are outlined where at centre stage is the ability to wait, to be surprised; to operate from the place of the unconscious, which by definition is a place of negativity, and to exercise a form of soft scepticism – ultimately, a mode of hospitality.

An Apocryphal Dictionary of Psychoanalysis will be of great use to psychoanalysts and psychoanalytic psychotherapists.

Giuseppe Civitarese, MD, PhD, is a training and supervising analyst (SPI, APsaA, IPA). He lives in Pavia, Italy. His books include *The Intimate Room: Theory and Technique of the Analytic Field*; *The Violence of Emotions: Bion and Post-Bionian Psychoanalysis*; *Truth and the Unconscious*; and *Sublime Subjects: Aesthetic Experience and Intersubjectivity in Psychoanalysis*.

Psychoanalytic Field Theory Book Series

S. Montana Katz & Giuseppe Civitarese
Series Editors

The Psychoanalytic Field Theory Book Series was initiated in 2015. The series publishes books on subjects relevant to the continuing development of psychoanalytic field theory. The emphasis of this series is on contemporary work that includes a vision of the future for psychoanalytic field theory.

Since the middle of the twentieth century, forms of psychoanalytic field theory emerged in different geographic parts of the world with different objectives, heuristic principles, and clinical techniques. Taken together they form a family of psychoanalytic perspectives that employs a concept of a bi-personal psychoanalytic field. The Psychoanalytic Field Theory Book Series seeks to represent this pluralism in its publications. Books on field theory in all its diverse forms are of interest in this series. Both theoretical works and discussions of clinical technique will be published in this series.

The series editors S. Montana Katz and Giuseppe Civitarese are especially interested in selecting manuscripts which actively promote the understanding and further expansion of psychoanalytic field theory. Part of the mission of the series is to foster communication amongst psychoanalysts working in different models, in different languages, and in different parts of the world. A full list of titles in this series is available at: www.routledge.com/Psychoanalytic-Field-Theory-Book-Series/book-series/FIELDTHEORY

An Apocryphal Dictionary of Psychoanalysis

Giuseppe Civitarese

Routledge
Taylor & Francis Group
LONDON AND NEW YORK

First published in English 2019
by Routledge
2 Park Square, Milton Park, Abingdon, Oxon OX14 4RN

and by Routledge
52 Vanderbilt Avenue, New York, NY 10017

Routledge is an imprint of the Taylor & Francis Group, an informa business

This book is a translation of a work previously published in Italian by Mimesis Edizioni as *Trasposizioni: Glossarietto di psicoanalisi* (Milan/Udine, 2017).

Translated by Luiza Dubicka.

British Library Cataloguing-in-Publication Data
A catalogue record for this book is available from the British Library

Library of Congress Cataloging-in-Publication Data
A catalog record has been requested for this book

ISBN: 978-0-367-14318-3 (hbk)
ISBN: 978-0-367-14321-3 (pbk)
ISBN: 978-0-429-03125-0 (ebk)

Typeset in Times New Roman
by Swales & Willis, Exeter, Devon, UK

To my patients

Everywhere I recognize transpositions

F. Nietzsche

Contents

Preface

Fragments of clinical vignettes, enigmatic objects, stray thoughts, projects, images, notes from readings, musings; but also, remarks on films and exhibitions, memories, episodes from daily life, summaries of papers to write, questions and doubts, obsessions: this here is a book of *transpositions*. Seen through the prism of my identity as a psychoanalyst, they were all born at moments when I had the impression of shining a little light on certain problems that arise in everyday work or on some obscure but fascinating points of theory. A trait common to these small epiphanies is, therefore, the intense relationship that links them to the experience of life. There is always an emotion in them: be it that of amusement, astonishment, gratitude, sadness, joy.

Small but not insignificant, at least not for the writer, they are there to be offered as gifts, *xenia*,[1] for the 'guests' of these pages, for the readers. If they mostly have to do with a psychoanalytical point of view, it is because for me psychoanalysis is not simply a profession but rather a path which I have chosen in my work in order to feel more human and more real, as well as to approach the mystery of what it means to be human, and so also that of the humanity of another person. After all, in a search which continues even subsurface, with a mixture of anxiety and pleasure, like in everyone, what comes back are moments of light and shadow of the relationship with the object which for the first time created the world for us.

Secondly, this is a book of imaginary conversations with some of my most-beloved authors. If in order to have a mind another mind is needed, then throughout life something new can only be born from fortunate encounters and moments. As well as to some analysts and philosophers, I also pay my tribute to the subtle and inspiring work of Roland Barthes, to his passion for the haiku and for aphoristic writing. A certain practice of intertextuality (be it in a general sense, between disciplines and different fields of knowledge; be it in a more specific sense, between different models of psychoanalysis), as well as attention to the use of quotations results from my innate curiosity and a long-standing interest in Walter Benjamin; while from Italo Calvino I get all the elements of a poetics of lightness and quickness.

Begun during a trip from Milan to Seattle, this little notebook was partly inspired by Giorgio Agamben's[2] book *Language and Death: The Place of Negativity*. During the outbound flight, while skimming through its wonderful but difficult pages, I was surprised to notice that the clouds outside had taken on a form of a vast expanse of ice flooded with a dazzling light but, thanks to a strange phenomenon, composed of many rectangles separated by deep and regular grooves, just like the ploughed and colourful fields that you see when you are about to land. This seemed to me an allegory of what Agamben was trying to do in dialogue with Hegel and Heidegger: to perimeter, with their help, the fields of the unsayable and the negative. After a couple of minutes, the shape of the clouds changed into that of a multitude of water lilies like those painted by Monet, but water lilies made of ice, and floating on the immense pond of the sky. Fields and water lilies which exist only in language and in the amazing possibility that language gives us to transpose all things.

For me psychoanalysis is precisely this ability to wait, to be surprised, to operate from the place of the unconscious, which by definition is a place of negativity, and to exercise a form of soft scepticism – ultimately, a mode of hospitality. The glossary thus expresses my style as an analyst and a person in treating mental suffering and gives a glimpse into the imaginary which nurtures it.

It is therefore an 'apocryphal' glossary because the entries are chosen on a personal basis and are often unconventional, and so for the most part do not correspond to the canon. But even in all their variety, an attentive reader will observe that they are like many tiles of a single mosaic. Is fragmentation not a figure of the freely associative trend of analytic discourse? In fact, the various terms are all linked by a few essential threads, the main one being the birth of the mind and the feeling of beauty in the relationship with the object; essentially an inquiry into the meaning of being.

Notes

1 See J. Derrida, 1997, *Of Hospitality*, Stanford, CA: Stanford University Press, 2000, p. 29: 'Herodotus said that Polycrates had concluded a *xenia* (pact) with Amasis and that they sent each other presents: *xenien sunethèkato*'.

2 G. Agamben, 1991, *Language and Death: The Place of Negativity*. Minneapolis, MN: University of Minnesota Press, 2006.

Foreword

Four monographs by Giuseppe Civitarese have already been translated into English for the prestigious New Library of Psychoanalysis Series. Now, this latest volume represents to some extent a 'summa' of his previous works, though one should say from the outset that the structure of the book is quite different. Readers will still find here a number of 'staple themes' of Giuseppe Civitarese's analytic thought: the aesthetic unconscious, narratology, post-Bionian field theory with its clinical ramifications/implications – and throughout, a constant and sensitive interest in all that (in art and everyday life, and in every analytic session) is 'rhythm'. A foundational rhythm of presence and absence, separation and at-one-ment, identity and difference, figure and background. Crucially, also, a rhythm whose successful modulation lies at the roots of our capacity to give emotional sense to our stories – or better still, to keep creating meaning through the narrations and representations that, more or less consciously, we produce at every given moment.

An integrated bodily awareness (an artistic awareness) of the affective meaning of rhythm breathes life into many of these pages, also infused by a sustained curiosity for the turns of meaning that psychoanalysis invariably presents to those who plunge into its depths of surprise and disquiet. Such a willingness to face the unknown, already familiar to Civitarese's readers, goes hand in hand with a passion for care. In Civitarese's theoretical frame of reference, psychoanalytic care is best understood as a process aimed at increasing the functions of the mind which, over time, will support patients in their gradual opening up to change and new experiences (of themselves). It is thus no coincidence that the book is dedicated 'to my patients', to whom Civitarese (in a touching poem entitled 'Lost and found') symbolically returns forgotten 'objects' left for some time in his office. With the discreet gracefulness of these lines, Civitarese alludes to one of the key tasks of an analytic treatment: that is, to offer patients through words – words that can finally replace concrete 'objects' – quotas of aliveness, thought, and creativity that were never developed, or possibly were somehow lost and never claimed back (speaking of creativity, one of the various objects in the 'lost and found' list is a guitar pick!).

The avowedly unsystematic and often delectably aphoristic structure of this volume sets it apart from the more traditionally academic books that preceded it. The same could be said of its tone, which one will find less restrained by the requirements of scientific prose. Instead, the voice readers will discover here has something of that elusive quality Italo Calvino called 'lightness' – a kind of mental mobility that is inspiring as it is contagious. Quoting Paul Valéry in his *Six Memos for the Next Millennium*, Calvino reminded us that the lightness one should aim for is not the quality of feathers, subject to the forces of winds and gravity, but the more solid virtue of birds: it is not, therefore, a passive quality, but the freedom of those who have become able to carry their own weight (the burden of having a mind) and for this reason now find it possible to look around, explore, take off. This sense of active, pleasurable lightness runs through all Civitarese's 'flashes' of analytic thought, which lend themselves well to a liberating experience of explorative, unsystematic reading.

Francesco Capello, School of European Culture and Languages (Modern Languages),
University of Kent, UK

A

A WOM*E*N. In the text of a session brought to supervision, a colleague writes about Ms. H., 'a wom*e*n' instead of 'a woman'. Somebody points out the error and so he realizes that what he is dealing with is not a single patient but a plurality of patients of various ages. In particular, the various versions of Ms. H. involved in obscure relationships, as she called them – that is in destructive sentimental ties. When Ms. H. tells her sadomasochistic stories, the analyst defensively connects them only to the material reality and does not make a link with a possible unconscious significance with respect to the analytical relationship in the here and now. For example, stressing the fact that Ms. H has a successful career, he highlights how much she is sought after by *headhunters*. In this, however, the group of colleagues immediately sees a figure in the analytic field. The analyst presenting the case realizes how at times he struggled to see in Ms. H. the little girl who at four years of age was still not able to talk. For example, instead of 'allowing' this little girl to metaphorically eat Nutella (one day when she mentions it), he pointed out that it is a mixture of fat and sugar. In short, he addresses the adult, chooses to focus the conflict, does not sufficiently welcome Ms. H.'s request to be nourished by the play and the intimacy of the analysis. By doing this, he fails to set the right level of communication and hinders the mental growth of the patient during the session. *Suddenly, the double meaning of the headhunter hologram in their relationship becomes clear.*

ABANDON. Anna Prohaska who sings Monteverdi's *Lamento della ninfa*.[1]

ABSENCE. In *L'Afrique fantôme* Michael Leiris[2] writes that being away from a woman can make one feel like living in the absent. Dissolved and vanished, she doesn't exist anymore as a separate body, but has become the space, the ghostly carcass through which one moves. I've always been struck by this sentence because it expresses very well the idea of spatialization of the object. Painting – especially Romantic painting inspired by the aesthetics of the sublime – is extraordinary for how it evokes in the landscape the shape of the object, which is often mysterious, enchanting and threatening all at the same time. What is brought to mind are paintings such as *The Mouth of a Cave* (1784) by Hubert Robert (Figure 1), or *At the Waterfall* (ca. 1850) by David Calypole Johnstone (Figure 2), or *A Mountain Pass* (1830) by William Turner,[3] all of which, as it were, previous 'versions' of the famous painting *The Origin of the World* (1866) by Gustave Courbet which decorated Lacan's house in Guitrancourt. The same is true for Camillo Sbarbaro's[4] poem *Esco dalla lussuria*, where the harsh relationship with the object is effectively transfigured in the ghostly landscape of the city. In this, the Kleinian contribution is everlasting. Every newborn can only continue to move in the mother's body. *Being born is an illusion.*

ABSTRACTION. Unforgettable pages in Heidegger's[5] book containing his seminars on Kant's first *Critique*, in particular those dedicated to the definition of the concept (unity in the multiplicity or 'representation of what is common to several ob-jects') and to the prerequisite for any thinking of the concept or sense of self. 'To abstract from' (*astrarre*) means simplifying, reducing a variety of beings to a common quality, eliminating differences and collecting similarities. In this way (through a sublimative transformation) you get the status of subject.

From a psychoanalytical point of view, the emotional unity between the mother and the infant is *a sort of primal abstraction* and occurs firstly in a purely sensory and indistinct dimension, and then in that of the emotional/sentimental space. Only at the end does it become possible to synthesize the concepts of logic. As Wittgenstein[6] writes: 'Knowledge is in the end based on acknowledgement'. The body that is lost in rising to the concept

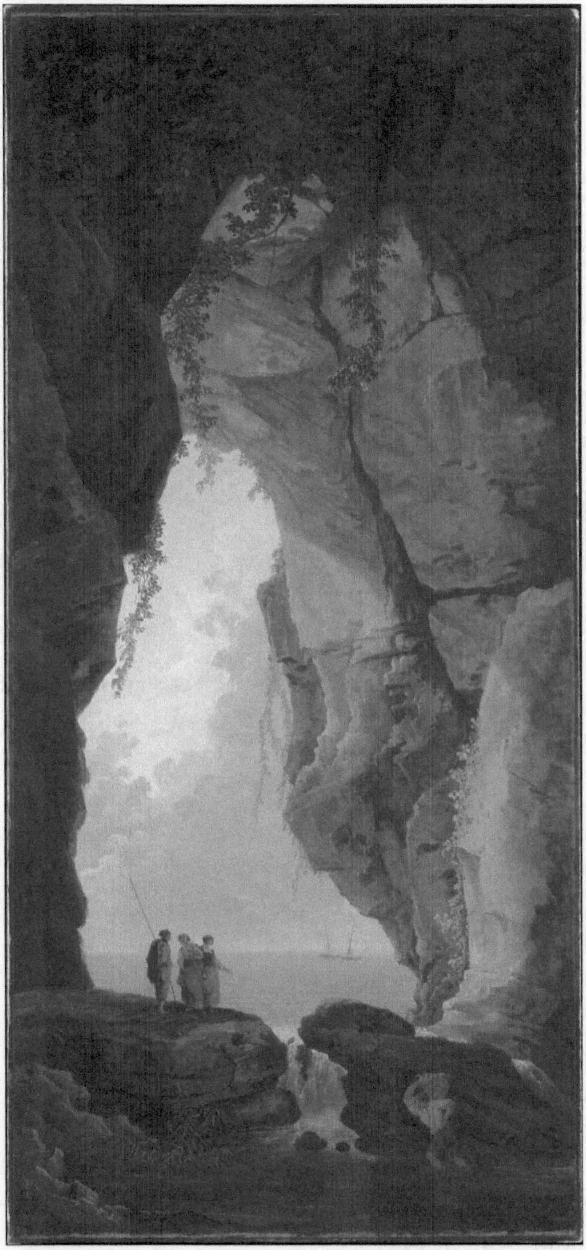

Figure 1 The Mouth of a Cave (1784) by Hubert Robert (French, Paris 1733–1808). Medium: oil on canvas. Dimensions: 68 3/4 × 31 1/4 in. (174.6 × 79.4 cm). Gift of J. Pierpont Morgan, 1917 to The Metropolitan Museum of Art, New York City, USA.

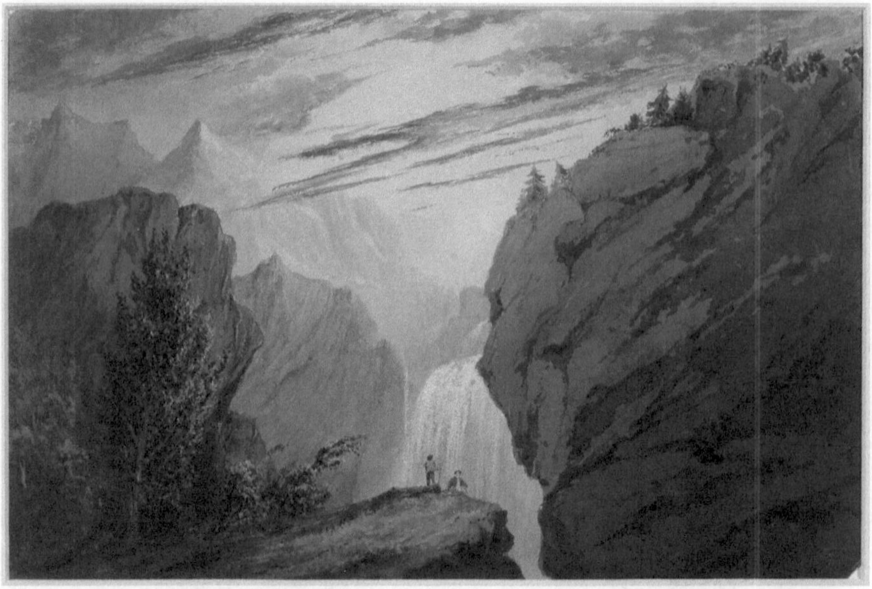

Figure 2 *At the Waterfall* (ca. 1850) by David Calypole Johnstone (American, Philadelphia, Pennsylvania 1799–1865 Dorchester, Massachusetts). Medium: watercolour, gum arabic, and gouache on off-white wove paper. Dimensions: 8 5/8 × 12 3/4 in. (21.9 × 32.4 cm). Gift of Mr and Mrs Stuart P. Feld, 1978 to The Metropolitan Museum of Art, New York City, USA.

is the body as a source of obscure and vague sensations. In this sense, to subjectify oneself does not mean to lose but *to take on* the body in the sense of adopting the necessary emotional categories, the 'sensible concepts' indispensable to life.

ADOLESCENCE. Winnicott and Ogden give us two valuable keys to understanding the adolescent. The former writes that unlike the child, the adolescent does not play with toys but with 'world affairs'.[7] The latter writes that in his infinite goodness God created the adolescent, otherwise it would be too painful to separate yourself from your children. In their brilliant simplicity, these two points offer a view of the adolescent as a fascinating being and help us to understand him (and to put up with him).

AESTHETIC CONFLICT. Winnicott's[8] review of Marion Milner's book, *On Not Being Able to Paint* contains an *ante litteram* interpretation of the Meltzerian concept of aesthetic conflict. Winnicott notes that creativity is born from the 'primary human predicament' that the infant faces: 'the non-identity of what is conceived of and what is to be perceived'. What does it mean? That to

> the objective mind of another person seeing from outside, that which is outside an individual is never identical with what is inside that individual. But there can be, and must be, for health […] a meeting place, an overlap, a stage of illusion, intoxication, transfiguration.

The first concept we have of life would have to do, in short, with the area of 'overlap' between the joy caused by the smiling face of the mother and the unsettling wonder about her true feelings. The psychoanalytic notion of the aesthetic conflict gives theoretical substance to the ingenious intuition expressed by Keats[9] in what are perhaps his most famous lines: '"Beauty is truth, truth beauty," – that is all/Ye know on earth, and all ye need to know'.

Winnicott[10] then offers a convincing interpretation of the meaning of the aesthetic experience:

> In the arts this meeting place is pre-eminently found through the medium, that bit of external world which takes the form of the inner conception. In painting, writing, music, etc., an individual may find islands of peace and so get momentary relief from the primary predicament of healthy human beings.

In the sense of harmony and in the pleasure that it inspires, the work of art would be, in brief, a promise of happiness (according to the Stendhalian definition of beauty). By offering an opportunity for identification between an emotion and an outer form that induces it, by analogy with the relationship with the breast, the aesthetic experience would nourish faith in the love of the object. If this possibility is prevented and the mother's duplicity and sphinx-like impenetrability have the upper hand, the consequences can be rather serious. Winnicott adds:

> When the mother's behavior does not correspond to the cathected internal mother image, the child does not experience frustration, unpleasure, or anger. What happens is that the child tends to lose the capacity to relate to objects. If the capacity to get angry is retained, things are not too bad.[11]

AESTHETIC EXPERIENCE. It has to do mainly with the rhythm. Every game of lines, colours, or sounds as a story of the intervals between moments of meeting and separation from the object. For Derrida,[12] it is the concept of the trace, a term that extends, or brings it back, to any perception the dialectics of identity and the difference of the system of language, a socially ordered deposit of signs. In the quotation that follows, this notion is contained in the two terms 'politically' and 'archive':

> In my opinion, there is trace since there is experience, that is, referring to the other, difference [*différance*], referring to something else, etc. So, wherever there is experience there is trace, and there is no experience without trace. So everything is trace, not only what I write on paper or what I log into a machine, but also by making this gesture I make a trace [...] Animals trace, every living being traces [...] There is no archive without trace, but not every trace is an archive to the extent that the archive requires not only a trace, but also that the trace is properly controlled, organized, politically under control.

AFFECTOLOGY. *How I Ended This Summer*[13] can be considered a film about a father–son relationship. In a meteorological station lost in a beautiful but inaccessible place in the Siberian Arctic, a young intern, and a more mature employee live together for some time. They spend their days visiting various instruments which measure the wind and water current speed, temperature and atomic radiation. Then they transmit the data via radio to a collection headquarters. The collection is often difficult because of the weather conditions. The man assumes a fatherly attitude towards the boy. He watches him furtively, nourishing some concerns about his diligence on the job or making sure he does not put himself in danger (white bears are a constant threat). At a certain point, seeing that he is not focused enough on his job, he reproaches him bitterly and urges him to cross the line between adolescence and adulthood. The boy, however, slowly moves towards paranoia. He imagines that in the past the man got rid of another employee because the latter failed to perform his duties.

The surprising aspect of the film is the beauty of the landscape which, mixed with its dangerousness, lends itself as a metaphor for the vicissitudes of any relationship where the two parties are deeply committed and where a strong bond of dependence is created. Collecting meteorological information becomes a metaphor for the continuous monitoring that we, consciously or unconsciously, all do in order to gather emotive signals in the field of relationships: an *affectology*.

AIRBAG. A charming advertisement by BMW aired a few years ago on France 2.[14] A newborn is being breastfed when, due to an abrupt movement, he is pulled away from the mother's breast only to bounce back softly onto it. At this point a voice explains the allegory: 'Rappelez-vous les sensations de votre premier airbag!' ['Remember the sensations of your first airbag!'].

ALLEGORY I. Following some of Benjamin's remarks and Derrida's deconstruction, Paul de Man re-emphasized the role of allegory with respect to that of the symbol. While the symbol would be directly linked to what it symbolized, in a way that seems to be natural, obvious, intrinsic to the thing itself, allegory comes back repeatedly to denounce the unbridgeable gap interposed between words and things.

Now, more than symbolic, the language of dream is an allegorical language, and in this it denounces the essential split that founds the subject. In essence, 'speaking about anything else' (in Italian 'parlare d'altro', i.e. literally 'speaking about the other') in allegory means speaking and being spoken by the Other. In this lies the originality of the Freudian interpretation of dream language: freeing it from a banal symbolic reading and placing it instead in the context of the dreamer's network of associations. In a way, with Freud the dreamer becomes the only authorized interpreter of his own dream.

In analysis, and especially in the post-Bionian model of the analytic field, whatever is said is seen under the sign of allegory, because *it (also) always speaks of the other*, like in dreams.

Whatever the subject, it is always a matter of negotiating the reciprocal distance in the analytical relationship.

In Freud, however, there is also a strong anchoring in history and in the theory of the traumatic causation of neurotic symptom. For this reason, the modernity of allegory is disquieting: because it requires giving up the reassuring fullness of the symbol and of its 'necessary' bond with the symbolized thing, which in this case is the bi-univocal correspondence between trauma and symptom.

ALLEGORY II. This is how Gershom Scholem[15] expresses the same basic idea on allegory:

> Allegory consists of an infinite network of meanings and correlations in which everything can become a representation of everything else, *but all within the limits of language and expression* … That which is expressed by and in the allegorical sign is in the first instance something which has its own meaningful context, but by becoming allegorical this something loses its own meaning and becomes the vehicle of something else … [However] the symbol [is] a form of expression which radically transcends the sphere of allegory. In the mystical symbol, a reality which in itself has, for us, no form or shape becomes transparent and, as it were, visible, through the medium of another reality which clothes its content with visible and expressible meaning … The thing which becomes a symbol retains its original form and its original content. It does not become, so to speak, an empty shell into which another content is poured; in itself, through its own existence, it makes another reality transparent which cannot appear in any other form. *If allegory can be defined as the representation of an expressible something by another expressible something, the mystical symbol is an expressible representation of something which lies beyond the sphere of expression and communication*, something which comes from a sphere whose face is, as it were, turned inward and away from us. A hidden and inexpressible reality finds its expression in the symbol … Where deeper insight into the structure of the allegory uncovers fresh layers of meaning, the symbol is *intuitively* understood all at once or not at all.

AMBIGUITY. The word 'ambiguity' is mostly used in its negative sense. Yet William Empson's[16] book on the seven types of ambiguity dates back to 1930. In it, ambiguity is defined as the possibility of simultaneously considering alternative views to interpret a text avoiding pure and simple misunderstandings. But the ability to realize the ambiguity of all things in the world and to tolerate it is exactly what, according to Ogden, analysts strive to promote in their patients. Being able to see things according to the simultaneous multiplicity of angles that is proper to the unconscious makes us feel truer and more real.

ANALYSIS VIA SKYPE. Seeing yourself on top of the other and the other on top of yourself.

ANALYST.

> My husband has stolen from me the best analyst in town … and what's more … who knows what he tells him about me! I should let him know that it's not true, that I'm not like anything he says about me … Are you aware of those people who write anonymous letters pasting the characters of the alphabet cut out from newspapers?!

ANAMNESIS. To be read as if all the characters and events were invented. In this way, the rhetorical, stylistic and content-related analysis of the text, seen from the point of view of the work of the poetic function of the unconscious (that is, as an expression of its capacity for *phanopeia* and *melopoeia*[17]), already provides a lot of useful information on the patient and the cure.

ANAMORPHOSIS. Whatever their value may be, clinical reports presented for supervision recount always the 'nightmare' of an analysis, expressing aspects which the analyst and the patient have not even imagined or 'dreamt' of in a personal or meaningful way. As I interpret the practice of supervision, therefore, it is not so much a vision from *above*, as it is a vision *with*. I consider supervision a method to integrate *with measure* and to accomplish the dream of the session, rather than to judge the quality of the analyst's work. Instead of reducing it to alleged latent thoughts, it is a way to develop the metaphor in order to finally find the meaningful image. It is like giving back to the vision the figure that has undergone the controlled transformation of anamorphosis. In this ingenious perspectival deformation of the subject, which we find in figurative art, it is in fact essential to find the precise point of view from which it recomposes itself and becomes intelligible.

ANGELS. Rilke's poetry is an invaluable contribution to contextualizing how the trauma and the precocity of mourning are at the origin of language and subjectivity, or of the loss of a 'pure' space and time. It also shows us how the aesthetics of the sublime, to which it represents an ideal introduction, can help us to redefine the concept of sublimation. Moreover, Rilke is the young but already accomplished poet with whom Freud claimed to have taken a walk and discussed the feeling of the beautiful, as he wrote in his 'On transience'.[18]

In the *Duino Elegies*[19] the human condition emerges by difference from the comparison, on the one hand with the animal and on the other with the angel. The human being is suspended between the animality of impulses or instincts ('The guilty blood/that even river-god') and the terribleness of the angel, of its perfection closed in on itself (of an ideal Ego?).

Not being a subject, the animal is not really opposed to any object. It is immersed in an undivided flow of sensations with nothing in front of it. It lives in a 'pure' time and space. Unlike the human being,

> Dumb creatures gaze with their whole vision out […] But never for a single day have we/Clear space before us, space wherein the flowers/Spring endlessly. The world, and still the world,/ Never a nowhere, blank, without negation;/Pure space, surveillance-free, in which we breathe,/To know most inwardly, and not to covet.[20]

In his commentary Péter Szondi[21] writes: 'The creature sees the open with full gaze because it does not see death. Only the eyes of man are turned backwards, out of the open, for they alone see death, for only man is conscious of death'. It is then that pure space becomes the world. On the contrary, animal knowledge is infinite because it is not limited by any 'no', because they have nothing in front of them. In Rilke's words: 'This is the meaning of our lot: to stand/Opposite; nothing more; forever opposite'.[22]

Likewise, in *The Infinite* by Leopardi – another example of a poem inspired by the principles of the sublime – the hedgerow that prevents you from seeing most of the horizon's remotest reaches[23] is what impedes you from watching 'the open', the element of nature which allegorizes the nature of humanity. It is the obstacle that forces men to live in an enclosed space of existence, is what hinders the sight lines in the finite nature of man, in the 'in front of' (*Gegenüber*), in the self-awarness that separates things.

The other, the opposite of animality – of the two poles that lay the foundation of the field of tension within which the subject can exist – is the angel. The angel is frightening because he is devoid of a body. Because he asks to renounce the body. Because he is a pure ideality. But for man not only being all-body, that is pure instinctiveness, but also giving up the body means dying. The angel, in itself terrible, is in fact a representation of death. This is true even if the tension towards what the angel represents is vital, because it emancipates (elevates) us from animality, but only as long as we don't reach it. In philosophical language, the angel is a stretching towards or an ascending, which we would call a being-towards-death. Here is a dramatic outline of what the frightening object evokes in the experience of the sublime.

To be human, then, means to oscillate continuously between these two extremes and never to give up on any of them. The angel's renouncing of the animality of the body is self-sufficiency, not needing the other. It is also a figure of a maternal face which is self-absorbed, ghostly, imperturbable, autonomous, that of a sphinx which is never available and therefore a figure of the trauma of the origins that perhaps the creative frenzy of sublimation attempts to cure.

Beware, the discourse on giving up the body is not abstract. We see it every day in our patients. The one that renounces the body lives an alienated, inauthentic life, cut off from its instinctive or emotional sources. The angel as opposed to animality – instead, the hysterical symptom of conversion is a process which transports 'down' to the body, expressing the need to claim it back – also represents language and the human ability to think.

For the same reason, just like pure space, so the 'pure continuance'[24] that lovers feel dissolving in each other is illusory; it entails the cost of giving up their sense of existing as separate subjects. However, only for a moment, it makes them feel like angels, elevates them, carries them towards the angels.

The main point of discourse is that we can never cut the instinctual roots from which our aspiration to become angels is born: becoming an angel means to die.

Instead, a place where the interweaving of corporeality and ideality is most successful is in dream, in poetry, and in all art in general. Unlike the poetry of the dream, however, the poetic word is closer to the angel. The dream has a similar quality, as it presupposes the conquest of a dream *space*, which is always a space of language – thoughts without the thinker come before thinking, words before dreams, being before entity – but it is clear that the poetic word, which is most tuned to the frequencies of the group, is virtually universal in a way that the 'private' dream can never be.

The dynamics of 'displacement that elevates' is summed up effectively by the concept of sublimation, where by displacement I mean distancing oneself from animality, from the place without the 'no'. Furthermore, you see that sublimation has and must have a limit, otherwise for the subject it would mean becoming an angel, and entering another type of pure space and time, opposite but coincident with that of the animal. Those who know how/are able to sublimate to levels of exceptionality, manage to combine both: 'instinctiveness' and 'perfection', id and super-ego, narcissism and socialism. Not only that, they also succeed in socializing their conquest. But you could also reverse the discourse, and say that the actual conquest *is* socializing and that the realization of a concrete object of art is only an instrument to achieve it; that the function expressed by form is more important than the content of the object itself. The necessary aspect of the materiality of the work means witnessing the presence of the body. At zero degree, then, it is true that sublimation is that of language, which entails the double mourning of the perfect coincidence of words with things on both sides of the body and of ideality.

The problem of sublimation is too often placed in extreme 'yes or no' terms, of either complete renunciation of the body or no renunciation at all, but it is essential to consider a quantitative or a balancing factor. For Freud, 'such sublimation is complete or incomplete, the analysis of character of highly gifted, especially of artistically disposed persons, will show a proportionate blending between productive ability, perversion and neurosis'.[25] The relationship between sublimation and creativity becomes clear, then, as an ideal equilibrium in the conflict between sublimation and its opposite or that which anchors us (and must anchor us) to the materiality of the body

ANIMA. Before visiting the violin museum in Cremona I did not know what the 'sound post' of this instrument was (but In Italian it is called 'anima', the same word for 'soul'). It is a small spruce cylinder about 6 mm in diameter placed inside the sound box between the top and the back plates. Its function is to transmit vibrations from one to the other and to help distribute the tension produced by the strings. The sound quality and timbral balance of the instrument depend on its correct positioning. *If the violin sounds bad, explains the guide, you can move the 'anima'/'soul' a few millimetres*. I don't know if there is a more poetic definition of analysis.

ANXIETY. Freud's[26] astonishing sentence in his 'Beyond the pleasure principle' when he writes that dreaming would help transform fright (*Schreck*) into anxiety (*Angst*). Fright is traumatizing because it catches us unprepared in the face of danger. Anxiety, on the other hand, operates as a shield because it anticipates danger and makes us vigilant. As Barthes[27] says:

> One rehearses a future catastrophe so as not to be completely powerless when it really does happen. Hence the hysterical character of anxiety: it is a *rehearsal* in the theatrical sense [...] Anxiety is an ec-stasy [*ec-stasy*] of the same intensity as a perceptual hallucination, a hallucination of danger.

APHASIA. An aphasic tension dominates all theoretical discourse in psychoanalysis, which is quite similar to that of a lover who cannot fully express his ineffable feeling for the adored object. Likewise, the ineffable shines through in many clinical accounts in the archaic rhetoric, the *pathos* of abysmal sufferings and the immersions into the world of psychosis.

ARCHAIC. A magic formula to be articulated when facing a serious case. Claim that you are in the presence of 'something very primitive or archaic'. The relief is immediate.

ASYMMETRY. If a character from the analytical field, for example the wolf from Little Red Riding Hood, is seen as a 'hologram' which results from the crossing of the patient's and the analyst's projective identifications, it means that it expresses a field *function*. At any given moment, the field is filled with emotions which we can attribute to the character of the wolf – and to its conduct. It would be wrong to assign responsibility for this exclusively to the patient or to the analyst, because then the field metaphor would be useless and we would be talking about the way two separate subjects influence one another. However, if the analyst identifies with the wolf character and brings the field symmetry back to a work asymmetry, it is not because he does not see it anymore as an intersubjective element, but because it is his duty to take responsibility for it. *Analysts are obsessed with happy endings*.

ATTENTION I. Intentional attention is a function of the Ego and hence it is only present after this agency of the mind has been established. Within certain limits it gives us the possibility to decide *how* to proceed: focusing either on the oneiric or on the rational poles of psychic life, either on the primary or the on the secondary process. The fact that within certain limits this can be done, however, is also proof that there is no point in maintaining such a clear distinction between the two regimes of mental functioning, as classical psychoanalysis dictates. The restriction of the field of consciousness allowed by attention squeezes into a fraction of a second the long phylogenetic process of the synthesis of concepts. Perhaps passing from the primary process to the secondary process simply means narrowing the picture of consciousness, maintaining in the foreground the psychic elements of a linguistic-conceptual order and keeping in the background those less 'distilled', images mostly, which by definition are more ambiguous.

ATTENTION II. Bion rejects the primary/secondary process dichotomy (which is why I write un/conscious: to give an idea of the continuity between the conscious and unconscious, like the two faces of a Möbius strip), and so do neurosciences.[28] Binary opposition should perhaps be reformulated as a *continuum* between the infinite and uncontrollable production of *sense* of the play of signifiers of language and of the non-verbal language of images, and the finite of linguistic concepts and of semantic or verbal *meaning*. Obviously, each extremity of the somato-psychic constitution of the human being contains its opposite. On the one hand, images make sense because the one contemplating them is the subject (a being endowed with self-consciousness); and on the other, the meaning of word fades in the semiotic sense of the linguistic signifier (either of the auditory body or of the written traces which convey them). The conscious and the unconscious are therefore in dialectical relation to one another. You cannot have one without the other. The key element of the passage or, better yet, of the *intensification* of one with respect to the other, in a sort of game between the figure and the background, is the intentional function of attention; the purely human ability to favour in communication, and in that private but always intersubjective communication that is thinking, a language that is sometimes more analogic and sometimes more digital. Attention allows us to determine how we prefer to face reality, whether with gestures, emotions and images or rather with words and concepts. It's a bit like choosing to see more with the fovea or with the peripheral part of the retina. One can say that attention expresses a capacity for psychic adjustment.

AURA. Walter Benjamin referred to it as the quality of uniqueness, irreproducibility, and individuality of the work of art. Ultimately, a mark of authenticity, a theophany. Linked to the concept of '*im*mediacy' (the absence of interposition of times, places, facts or people) pursued with various tools and outcomes by all models of psychoanalysis, the aura of the *here and now* ('a strange web of space and time'[29]) would guarantee the truth of the facts (of O's transformations) of the analysis. This would be a *synchronic* immediacy, but there exists also a *diachronic* immediacy or, in other words, a 'narrative intimacy' given by the implicit enhancement of the story shared by the couple. In the interpretation process it functions as a test bed for interpretation.

AUTHENTICITY. The theme of authenticity is typically philosophical. Heidegger explains it as the inseparable link between language and finiteness. In psychoanalysis, however, it comes up in the Winnicottian distinction between the false and true self. In Bion, instead, in the concept of the truth drive,[30] in the dialectic between truth and lie and in dichotomy of being (O) and knowing (K).

AVOIDING (SOMEONE). It's the last session of the day. I'm very tired. I had to withstand unusual tensions since that morning. I open the door and am surprised to see a patient I was not expecting. For an instant I remain bewildered and do not shake her hand. After a fraction of a second I 'wake up' from my inertia. I stretch out my hand and apologize, giving her some generic reason. Slowly, afterwards, the scene comes back to me, charged with possible meanings. For a few sessions with this patient I was being careful to establish a little more distance. For a time I felt a little too involved and she pointed it out to me. Some of my too 'fatherly' or 'professor-like' comments about a certain problem at her workplace left little room for other important things. The scheme was 'I'll be as you'd like me to be'. By not shaking her hand, I was unconsciously expressing this still obscure intuition through action. Resentful, I replicated her behaviour in turn, but from another perspective, the 'as you want me' (that is, detached). In fact – but I understood this only after a while – we were functioning on the basis of a double misunderstanding: on her side she was ignoring the sense of my 'fatherly' investment, on my part, that of her contestation.

Notes

1 www.youtube.com/watch?v=XHRjvK9syQc (Accessed: July 8, 2018).
2 M. Leiris, 1934, *L'Afrique fantôme*. Paris: Gallimard, 1988.
3 www.tate.org.uk/art/artworks/turner-a-mountain-pass-d25213 (Accessed: June 13, 2016).
4 C. Sbarbaro, 2001 [1914], *Pianissimo*. Venezia: Marsilio.
5 M. Heidegger, 1997 [1973], *Phenomenological Interpretation of Kant's 'Critique of Pure Reason'*. Bloomington, IN: Indiana University Press, p. 153.
6 L. Wittgenstein, 1969, *On Certainty*. New York: J. & J. Harper Editions, p. 378. See also fragment 528, p. 71: 'And in spite of this: if someone asked me what the colour was called in German and I tell him, and now he asks me "are you sure?" – then I reply "I *know* it is; German is my mother tongue"'.
7 D. W. Winnicott, 1989, *Psycho-Analytic Explorations*. Cambridge, MA: Harvard University Press, p. 62.

8 *Ibid.*, p. 391.
9 J. Keats, 1900, *The Complete Poetical Works of John Keats*. Boston, MA; New York: Houghton Mifflin Harcourt, p. 235.
10 Winnicott, *Psycho-Analytic Explorations*, cit., p. 391.
11 *Ibid.*, p. 472.
12 J. Derrida, 2016 [2013], *Pensare al non vedere. Scritti sulle arti del visibile (1979–2004)*. Milano: Jaca Book, pp. 131–132.
13 A. Popogrebski (director), *How I Ended This Summer*, Russia, 2010.
14 www.dailymotion.com/video/x39uj3 (Accessed: July 7, 2018).
15 G. Scholem, 1961, *Major Trends in Jewish Mysticism*. New York: Schocken Books, pp. 26–27 (emphasis added). I thank Avner Bergstein for this quote.
16 W. Empson, 1966, *Seven Types of Ambiguity*. New York: New Directions.
17 E. Pound, 1991, *ABC of Reading*. London: Faber & Faber, p. 37.
18 S. Freud, 1957 [1915], 'On transience', *The Standard Edition of the Complete Psychological Works of Sigmund Freud*, vol. 14. London: The Hogarth Press.
19 R. M. Rilke, 1931 [1923], *Duineser Elegien: Elegies from the Castle of Duino*, translated by V. & E. Sackville West. London: Hogarth Press, p. 30.
20 *Ibid.*, pp. 89–91.
21 P. Szondi, 1995 [1975], *Le 'Elegie duinesi' di Rilke*. Milano: *SE*, p. 71.
22 Rilke, *Duineser Elegien*, cit., p. 90.
23 G. Leopardi, *The Infinite*, translated by Henry Reed. *Listener*, 43, no. 1113 (May 25, 1950), p. 924.
24 Rilke, *Duineser Elegien*, cit., p. 26.
25 S. Freud, 1962, *Three Contributions to the Theory of Sex*. New York: Dutton, p. 94.
26 S. Freud, 1920, 'Beyond the pleasure principle'. *SE*, vol. 18, pp. 1–64.
27 R. Barthes, 2007, *Il discorso amoroso. Seminario a l'École Pratique des Hautes Études 1974–1776, seguito da Frammenti di un discorso amoroso (inediti)*. Milano-Udine, Italy: Mimesis, pp. 429–430.
28 See D. Westen, 1999, 'The scientific status of unconscious processes: Is Freud really dead?', *Journal of the American Psychoanalytic Association*, 47:1061–1106.
29 W. Benjamin, 1955, *The Work of Art in the Age of its Technical Reproducibility and Other Writings*. Cambridge, MA: Harvard University Press, 2008, p. 285. See also: G. Civitarese, 2016, 'Truth as immediacy and unison: A new common ground in psychoanalysis? Commentary on essays addressing "Is truth relevant?"', *Psychoanalytic Quarterly*, 85:449–501.
30 J. S. Grotstein, 2004, 'The seventh servant: The implications of a truth drive in Bion's theory of "O"', *International Journal of Psychoanalysis*, 85:1081–1101. On this issue, see also G. Civitarese, 2013, 'Bion's Grid and the truth drive', *The Italian Psychoanalytic Annual*, 7:91–114.

B

BABEL. The image of language confusion is often evoked to negatively depict the state of the art in psychoanalysis. There would be too many psychoanalyses pointlessly searching for a common ground. I wonder if a way of conceptualizing this issue cannot be analogous to how we think about the disciplined use of intuition. The various models or theories would represent multiple and simultaneous points of view on the psychic life. Rather than seeing them from the reductionist perspective of technology or science, they could be seen from the perspective of poetic ambiguity. There would be plural and reasonable visions of the unconscious elaborated by the collective mind. In clinical work, of course, these different 'visions' should then be traced back to a necessary principle of theoretical and technical consistency. Having in the background the familiarity of different models, even if somehow 'incommensurable', not only does not affect the possibility of working in a non-banal and confusingly eclectic way, but can even give perspective to the choices that are then adopted and that it is *necessary* to adopt. In fact, in psychoanalysis artistic-intuitive moments coexist with more scientific-practical ones. Even in this, it qualifies itself, as is the case with Heidegger's concept of authentic thinking, as a 'restless to and fro between (*zwischen*) yes and no', a being 'suspended as it were between (*zwischen*) the two'.[1]

BEAUTY. A. tells me:

> I often dream of dying. I'm in my house in my favourite room. I contemplate the various furniture around me. Then I think, "But is it possible, now that I have finally decorated my room with the things I like the most, that I have to die?"

You find the same inspiration in the profound feeling of indignation which powerfully propels Philip Roth's eloquent and moving narrative ('the most beautiful word in the English language: "Indig-*na*-tion!"'[2] he writes in his novel of the same name). Sometimes a thought came upon me, while I was immersed in some place of overwhelming beauty, for example in Sardinia, but also in urban settings, in Rome, in New York …: 'People die here too?! It should not be allowed!' So, disturbing by definition, the anguish caused by the consciousness of the transience of all things weasels its way into the heart-wrenching feeling of beauty and therefore into that of the fullness of life. The beauty of the world, which we cannot do without, especially that which reaches the height of the sublime, is always a *painful* beauty. As in Leypold's (Figure 3) or in Ehrensvärd's painting (Figure 4), always like wanderers in the storm or at best watching it as if at sea from the shore.

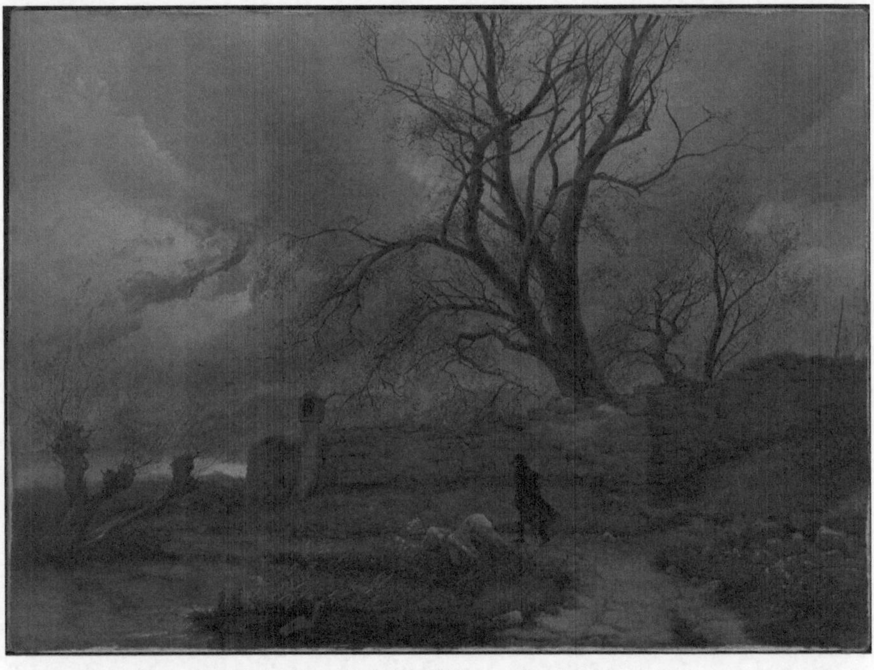

Figure 3 *Wanderer in the Storm* (1835) by Julius von Leypold (German, Dresden 1806–1874 Niederlößnitz). Medium: oil on canvas. Dimensions: 16 3/4 × 22 1/4 in. (42.5 × 56.5 cm). Catharine Lorillard Wolfe Collection, Wolfe Fund, 2008.

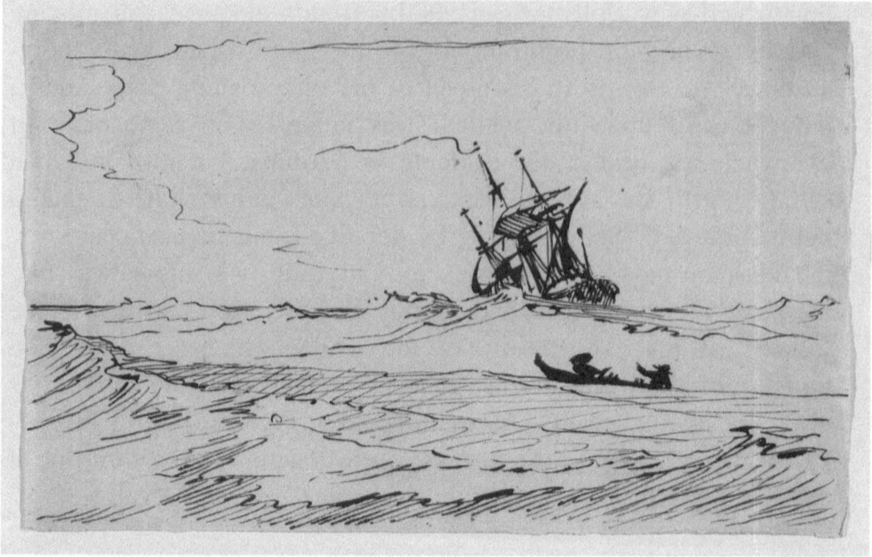

Figure 4 A Storm at Sea with a Large Ship and a Small Boat with Two Figures (1765–1800) by Car August Ehrensvärd (Swedish, 1745–1800). Medium: pen and black ink. Dimensions: Sheet: 8 1/4 × 13 1/16 in. (21 × 33.1 cm). The Elisha Whittelsey Collection, The Elisha Whittelsey Fund, 2014.

BENJAMIN. I have always been fascinated by the 'intertextual' and eclectic figure of Walter Benjamin: long before I was even able to understand anything he wrote. As with some books that have been bought but never read, books which have a secret life on the shelves of our library and which exert an influence on us nevertheless (U. Eco), so we sometimes choose figures that, while remaining long inaccessible, live as reassuring presences, and somehow inspire us. With Benjamin, however, from the very beginning, what stuck in my mind was his characterization of a painting as something that, unlike a photograph (which resembles, rather, thirst-quenching water), one does not ever tire of contemplating (the difference between need and desire?). Similarly, I was struck by the annotation in his essay on Leskov focusing on how central the death of the protagonist is in a tale or in a novel, as if it were the very last act which gave meaning to the whole and which moved the reader's curiosity.

BERGMAN. *I have a dream about being questioned during the exam to become a training analyst by two nearly-one-hundred-year-old examiners, with wrinkly loose skin. They speak to me in a foreign language and I do not understand the questions. In the dream, I think that these are not the real members of my commission and that they have found a way to reject me.*

It's my own *Wild Strawberries*-like dream.[3] The mind transforms the anxiety of the examination into 'poetic' images, and it also gives me useful guidance on how to introduce myself – without letting down my guard – and how to take into account the rigidity of psychoanalytic institutions and their inclination to dogmatism.

BODY-TEXT. It would take too long to retrace the story of how psychoanalysis engaged with the body from the beginning: from the hysterical symptom (the classical expression of the talking body) to the mute body of the alexithymic disorder.

About the body itself, the one studied by biology and anatomy, psychoanalysis cannot say anything because it does not know anything. Psychoanalysis deals with the body-as-signifier, the body-as-text. The body that interests psychoanalysis is the body that communicates. How? With words, with the body of words and in a non-verbal way with posture and gestures. As a result, we never have to deal with a natural body, out of the symbolic context in which we are inevitably immersed even before birth. That's why the psychoanalytic unconscious has nothing to do with that of neurosciences.

Yet the limits within which the body speaks remain opaque. If it can be easy to understand the reason behind a stutter or a blush, an extrasystole or a fainting, what can be said about the lesions we order in the diagnostic categories of psychosomatics? Why not adopt the radical theories of Judith Butler, who boldly subordinates the anatomy to culture?

In psychoanalysis, therefore, we find ourselves faced with two opposing views: the body as an absolute limit – (and it must be said that in Karl Jaspers's psychiatry delusion also marked the unpassable border of the incomprehensible, and then this area was re-annexed by Freud to the comprehensible) – and the body completely textualized.

BOOKHOUSE (CASALIBRO). Novels ask us to suspend our usual disbelief and to surrender to fiction. Where we see letters and words we imagine homes, people, adventure. Gabriele D'Annunzio's *The Shrine of Italian Victories*, the estate in Gardone Riviera overlooking Lake Garda where he lived his last years, invites us to go the other way: to see letters and words from the pages of a novel in walls, rooms, and objects. The entirely imaginary adventure of Mr Kugelmass, a character created by Woody Allen,[4] who, having failed his analysis, is sent by a magician into the pages of *Madame Bovary* because he fell in love with the protagonist, along with *The Shrine of Italian Victories* becomes an experience actually lived.

BOUVARD AND PECUCHET. Small contribution to a psychoanalytic dictionary of clichés, chic ideas and various nonsense: 'Freud had already said it', 'Why call this thing psychoanalysis?', 'There is a certain risk of deviation here', 'What happens to [as appropriate: the subject, the unconscious, the trauma, the Reality, the Past …]?!', 'It's too difficult', with another possible variant 'It's too easy … '. The proper tone to correctly pronounce these phrases should be between smug-prophetic and concerned, and it should never lack a certain emphasis, as of one who is quite pleased with himself.

BREAKDOWN. In his famous article on the fear of breakdown, Winnicott[5] interprets it as if it had already happened, Ogden[6] as if it did not happen because it was not experienced, and Barthes[7] as a repetition of a future catastrophe.

Notes

1 M. Heidegger, 1966 [1959], *Discourse on Thinking*. New York: Harper & Row, p. 75.
2 P. Roth, *Indignation*. New York: Houghton Mifflin Harcourt, 2008, p. 95.
3 I. Bergman (director), *Wild Strawberries*, Sweden, 1957.
4 W. Allen, 1977, 'The Kugelmass episode', *The New Yorker*, May 2.
5 D. W. Winnicott, 1989, *Psycho-Analytic Explorations*. Cambridge, MA: Harvard University Press, p. 62.
6 T. H. Ogden, 2014, 'Fear of breakdown and the unlived life', *International Journal of Psychoanalysis*, 95:205–223.
7 R. Barthes, 2007, *Il discorso amoroso. Seminario a l'École Pratique des Hautes Études 1974–1776, seguito da Frammenti di un discorso amoroso (inediti)*. Milano-Udine, Italy: Mimesis, pp. 429–430.

C

CADUCITY. Freud's brief essay 'On transience' can be read as the negative of the *Duino Elegies*. In a nutshell, 'On transience' contains a theory of aesthetic experience that is alternative – or, if you will, complementary – to that of sublimation. This short text was written in 1915 when Freud was invited to contribute to a volume dedicated to Goethe. Perhaps it is for this reason that Freud starts his discourse by evoking the figure of a young but already established poet with whom he discussed beauty during a mountain trip in the Dolomites. The poet's identity is not known with certainty, but it is likely that it was Rilke. The poet expresses to Freud his sorrow for the ephemeral nature of all things, in particular, of beauty and art. Freud,[1] on the contrary, argues that the transience of beautiful things does not demean but rather elevates their value, giving them 'a fresh charm'. When, instead, transience produces boredom or rebellion – here two figures of depression and delusion – it seems to be that we are in the presence of pathological reactions. The non-pathological response would be the processing of grief.

Mourning in itself is an enigma, Freud explains. You don't see why it is so difficult to detach oneself from the lost object, especially when a new object is available. Another point of his argument in response to the poet's pessimism is that things have no value in themselves but only in relation to human sensitivity. It would not make sense, so to speak, to complain about the transience of beauty in itself, regardless of who will react to it. Freud then mentions the possible destructive but inexorable effects of the 'geological eras'. It is easy to interpret this statement also in reference to the coming war. Ultimately 'On transience'theorizes the aesthetic experience as a successful work of mourning and, vice versa, the work of mourning as analogous to the psycho-physical fullness of the aesthetic experience.

Therefore, if we cannot safely say that it was Rilke – and Andreas Lou Salomé: the figure of the 'silent friend' in the text – there are enough coincidences to lead us to read some of the aesthetic themes expressed by the Prague poet in his *Duino Elegies* in the light of Freud's text.

CAESURA. In a short text written at the end his life, Bion[2] summarizes the only principle of method to which he seems to have always been faithful: systematically practising the art of doubt and deconstructing all the binary oppositions on which classical psychoanalysis founds meaning. In his case, the summary formula of this agenda is 'transcending the caesura'. The art of doubt can be practised by embracing a radically phenomenological method, starting from the immediate data of experience, and setting aside the rest. In Bion, the Cartesian 'I think therefore I am' is, on the one hand, paying attention to what is happening here and now as immediacy and is therefore the measure of truth, and, on the other hand, putting at the centre of inquiry the development of the mechanism for thought. However, Bion can, so to speak, stand on the shoulders not only of Descartes but also of Kant and Husserl (and be inspired by the latter's famous 'We must go back to the "things themselves" [*Wir wollen auf die "Sachen selbst" zurückgehen*]'[3]). This is why, unlike the former, he can say that the formulation of the *cogito* should be corrected to 'I lie therefore I am': because after the Copernican revolution operated by Kant we are all now aware that the thing-in-itself (or reality) is unattainable and that, paradoxically, thinking is always, in one way or another, lying.

CENTRAL STATION. Since they opened a Bistro and a Feltrinelli bookshop at Milan Central Station, travelling by train (provided it is a Frecciarossa) has become quite pleasant. My first stop is the Bistro coffee shop, my second stop the bookshop. Precisely, in the following order: first, the poetry shelf, then psychology (with a glance at critical theory just opposite), and lastly philosophy. As you can see, the 'central station' is still psychoanalysis.

CHAGALL. In Chagall's painting *The Nude over Vitebsk*[4] (1933) the landscape of a city is topped by a huge sensual nude of a woman seen from behind. The object, as Freud writes, is our first home.

Chagall's painting suggests that, unconsciously, it remains such forever. Never again will there be access to nature except through the filter of the human.

In other subjects, Chagall shows microscopic scenes inside the head or above the head of animals or people (for example a small rabbi over the head of a rabbi figure), evoking the phantasmagoria of images that come alive in the theatre of the mind.

CHARACTER. In the dream of the session everything is transfigured. Any scene is read in allegorical terms. People, things, and even abstract entities become the protagonists of a narrative fiction. Transformed into characters in the analyst's receptive listening, but confirmed to the patient as real, they are used as potholders to touch emotions at the white heat without getting burnt. If, for example, anger is not *im*mediately mine or the patient's but Chiara's or Lucia's, one keeps a distance that does not interrupt the dream or the film of the session. Sometimes, however, you can effectively play the card of narrative metalepsis. This is what happens when, for example, a transference interpretation is given and a short circuit between non-logically connected worlds is created.

CINDERELLA. If the spectator did not know about the previous metamorphosis, he would think that it is when the carriage turns back into a pumpkin that Cinderella begins to hallucinate. From this one can see the importance of context: 'There is no outside-text', says Derrida.[5]

COLD. A. keeps flinging so much rage towards me that once I'm left alone I continue to shake for about ten minutes. It would appear that it is because of the cold outside and the fact that the heating has not been turned on yet, but perhaps it is even more due to my efforts to keep calm. I think there must be a terrible frost inside of her.

COMICS. To get the qualification to practise, an analyst should demonstrate a knowledge of, in order of relevance, at least *Peanuts, Calvin & Hobbes, B.C.* and *The Fusco Brothers*. After these you could have *Zerocalcare, Dastardly and Muttley, Professor Balthazar*, and *Colt*. At one point or another they all came in handy in my clinical work to talk to the patient in a simple manner and not in a cold or abstract way.

CONCEPT. The concept is an example of a container. We read in Heidegger:[6]

> Kant says: 'Every concept contains *in* itself a multiplicity, to the extent that it agrees but also to the extent that it is different.' In the multiplicity contained in a concept there lies the unity of a unanimous agreement *and* at the same time the manifold as different [...] The *wherein* the many objects agree is a *unifying one* [*Einiges*] and selfsame. And only as this one, as this definite *unity*, can it encompass a many and contain many within itself – only thus can it be common to the many and be contained in them.

Elsewhere, to say 'concept' Heidegger[7] uses expressions like 'seize-in-one', 'grasp-together-in-one', 'put together the manifold'; for example, the concept of 'treeness [*Baumhafte*]' derives from many trees; and then, as usual, he throws out a surprising phrase:

> but the concept of the 'tree' does not grow anywhere [...] every concept is a 'mere' concept, never something 'objective', and therefore *only* 'subjective', something that comes to exist in the human 'subject'; somewhere in the head or elsewhere, and therefore activity with 'concepts' and 'mere concepts' is like getting-lost 'distant from reality' with no 'proximity to life' [*eine wirchlichkeitsferne Verirrung ohne Lebensnähe*].

However, only a few lines down, he denies that the concept is a 'mere representation' and recalls its nature of 'taking in the essence [*Griff in the Wesentliche*]'.

What is represented here is the dual nature of the concept: not a 'mere' concept, but also not 'the being itself', rather 'the convincing bond between man and things, and between man and man'. But how can we forget the disquieting characterization of the concept flashed before the reader first, even just to be then discarded, the 'getting-lost [*Verirrung*]'? Perhaps more than philosophers, analysts do know how one can get lost in abstraction. For example, Winnicott speaks of 'escape into the intelligence' and of a 'false self, living through a mind or intellectual life which has become separated off from the psyche-soma'.[8]

In another text, 'The origin of the work of art', Heidegger[9] leads us onto the path of violence that thought can exert on the real:

> what is the use of a feeling, no matter how certain, if the word belongs to thought alone? Yet perhaps what, here and in similar cases, we call feeling or mood is more rational – more perceptive, that is – than we think; more rational, because more open to being than that 'reason' which, having meanwhile become *ratio*, is misdescribed as rational.

Reflection/abstraction or the 'function of unificaton' reduces the multiple to one; *unites* it. Elsewhere Heidegger[10] adds: 'reflection functions in the manner of unifying; it reveals the one as possible basis for the agreement of the many, so that with the aid of the unity so obtained a relation to the many is explicitly constituted'. It is difficult not to read these passages in view of Bion's concepts of 'psychoanalytic function of personality' – which we can understand, similarly to the reflective function of the mind, as a spontaneous activity of thinking – and then of a unison/*at-onement*, 'common sense'. What these psychoanalytic concepts add to the philosophical speculation is the fine and empirically based analysis of the indubitable intersubjective dimension in which the reflective function can only be born and develop. For its part, philosophical inquiry helps us to grasp the complexity of the concept of 'unison', now raised to a principle of therapy in post-Freudian psychoanalysis. The object performs the task of ordering the multiple representations of the infant into 'concepts'. In this sense, the prototype of a 'concept' is the area where the cheek and the breast face each other and which offers soothing sensations.[11] But then is metaphor (or Freud's condensation) also not a sort of concept at its zero degree? Does it not consist in the identification of a common-being to two different terms? It is important to realize how the *unison* (being-one) is always in fact a finding of a unity in diversity. There are many ways in which the unity of a union is determined, that is, the unity in which the concept contains the being-common is generated. In analysis, whenever one interprets transference, he reduces the multiple to a unity, preforms the act of synthetizing the 'understanding *in one*',[12] abstracts from the differences to focus on an essential being-common to two different situations: one present and the other past.

CONDENSATION. Ezra Pound:[13] 'Great literature is simply language charged with meaning to the utmost possible degree'. Then just below he notes: 'Dichten = condensare [condensing]'.[14] Curiously Pound uses the Italian for to 'condense', the verbal form of the word 'condensation' chosen by Freud to indicate, along with 'displacement', one of the fundamental mechanisms of the dream rhetoric. What is noteworthy here is the identification *dreaming* = *writing poetry.*

CONFUSION. Though tolerable, the reintrojection of a split and projected part of one's personality generates confusion. One goes back to the preceding stage of the *failure* of confusion as a defence against anxiety. However, if in the meantime the ability to tolerate anxiety – so *before* it becomes desperation – has increased, the confusion is mitigated, it is only temporary, and is proof of the beginning of an effective process of reintegration.

COVER. For my third book in the Routledge *New Library of Psychoanalysis*, an old drawing by my son G. (Figure 5) from when he was little, because it evokes the play and the magical world of dreams.

CREAM. The 'new' therapeutic factors in an acronym: play the Greek **C**horus, use the **R**êverie to dream the session, name the **E**motions, pay attention to h**A**llucinosis, suggest happy **M**etaphors.

CRISIS. As in any couple's life, so in analysis there are moments of crisis. This is what Anna feared, and that is why she immediately dreamed about a movie entitled *Amabili resti* [*The Lovely Bones*]. The imperative '*Ama* [Love]!' doesn't need an explanation. As opposed to the stolen letter in Poe's famous story, the invocation is hidden only to be brought to light. Inverting the order of words gives us *Resti amabili*: 'You remain loveable', with or without an exclamation point, that is either as an injunction or as a simple enunciation. By joining the two words, from *Restiamabili*, you get '*Restiam[o] (am)abili*' ('We remain loveable'/'Let's remain loveable'); and, be it '*amo*' ('I love [you]') or, other than the already seen '*ama*' ('Love [me]!', '[She/he] loves [you]'). Lastly what is also contained in 'am[abil]i' is '*ami*', which means both 'You love [me]' and 'hooks or lures'.

CRONUS. For Bion, the symbol is a *no-thing* that is born of the absence of the *thing* (the object), but of which there remains a trace, more precisely, of the place where it used to be but where it no longer exists. Such an affirmation, however, is partial and

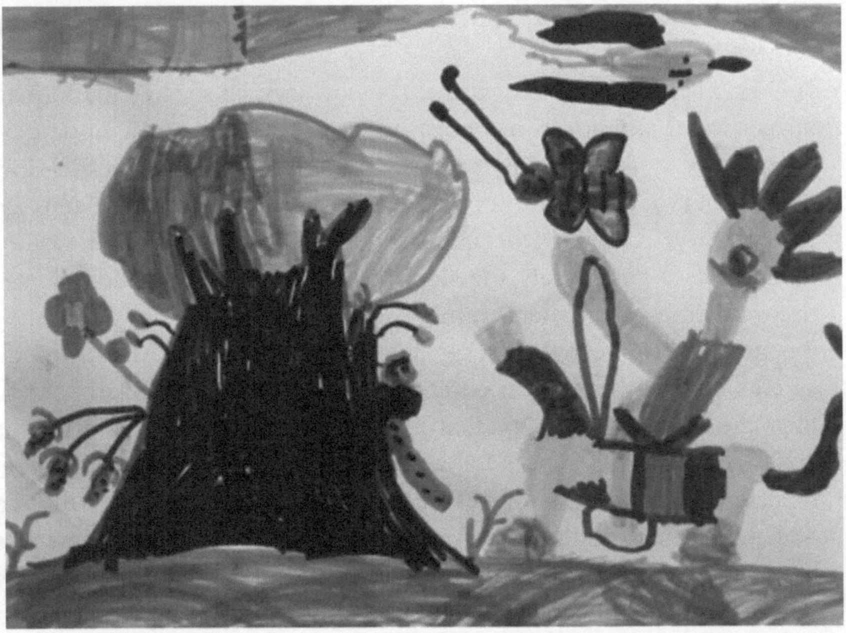

Figure 5 G.'s drawing.

leaves us with the impression that for a better understanding of what we are doing we need to bring in a new actor. It is not enough to say 'absence'. Absence must be *tolerable* – a too-absent-a-mother would become a dead mother, where the adjective expresses the idea that the ability to symbolize is a function of the *duration* of absence.

Looking a little closer, the no-thing could then be split into two elements: in the *no-breast* or *no-penis*, which Bion depicts with the geometric marks of the point and the line. That is to say that conversely the *thing* is composed of *breast* and *penis*, namely, of an object (the 'mother' or whoever acts as one) and of a paternal function, a third one, that it must have in itself and which regulates its distance to the infant: not too close because it would become 'incestuous' and not too far because it would fail to overcome its anxiety, leaving it to the cold and the loneliness of an infinite space. By splitting the *no-thing* into two elements we have two coordinates to consider: the point (the presence of the object and its trace) on the one hand and the separating or gathering element of the line, i.e. of *time*. And here is the missing actor: Cronus.

CYCLOTHYMIA. The cyclic nature of moods can be seen as the forever unsuccessful attempt to reconnect the mind and the body. In depression, the body is so heavily at the centre of the scene that it can slow down motor activity and turn off mimicry and thinking. In mania, on the contrary, everything becomes airy, the cancerous proliferation of thought loses completely the sight of the body and its needs. Sometimes severe manic patients remain awake for days and days, as if they did not need to recover energy with sleep. It is as if during mood swings the body-acrobat tried at times to catch the head-acrobat and then the opposite. The cyclicity could be a symptom and also, as always, a partial solution for a basic disjunction between different representations of the object and different relationships with the object. In other words, what you see, impressed in these remarkable metamorphosis as watermarks, are the vicissitudes with the primary object. The cue comes from Barthes.[15] In the paragraph dedicated to the term 'rhythm', he mentions the cyclicity of the mood of lover, virtually a manic-depressive in perpetual oscillation between triumphant moments of narcissistic flashes, when one sees confirmation in the love of the object, and depressive moments when one despairs over the love of the object. From this angle, evocative figures of cyclothymia, seen here as an example of a state of de-personalization of the subject, are the characters in Chagall's paintings who are depicted upside down or float in the air with their head separated from the body. For example, *Homme à la tête verte flottante ou personnage flottant*.

Notes

1 S. Freud, 1957 [1915], 'On transience', *The Standard Edition of the Complete Psychological Works of Sigmund Freud*, vol. 14. London: The Hogarth Press, p. 306.
2 W. R. Bion, 1981, 'Caesura', in F. Carrao, ed., *Il cambiamento catastrofico*. Torino: Loescher, pp. 79–99.
3 E. Husserl, 2001 [1900], *Logical Investigations*. London: Routledge, p. 168.
4 www.katarte.it/2014/09/marc-chagall-volare-dalla-russia-tra-le-fiabe-le-magie/chagall-nudo/ (Accessed: June 1, 2018).

5 J. Derrida, 1976 [1967], *Of Grammatology*. Baltimore, MD: Johns Hopkins University Press, p. 158.
6 M. Heidegger, 1997 [1973], *Phenomenological Interpretation of Kant's 'Critique of Pure Reason'*. Bloomington, IN: Indiana University Press, pp. 155–156.
7 M. Heidegger, 2014 [2009], *Pensieri–guida. Sulla nascita della metafisica, della scienza contemporanea e della tecnica moderna*. Milano: Bompiani, pp. 107–111.
8 D. W. Winnicott, 1989, *Psycho-Analytic Explorations*. Cambridge, MA: Harvard University Press, p. 467.
9 M. Heidegger, 2002, 'The origin of the work of art', in: J. Young and K. Haynes (eds and trans), *Off the Beaten Track*. Cambridge: Cambridge University Press, p. 7.
10 Heidegger, 1997 [1973], *Phenomenological Interpretation*, cit., p. 162.
11 T. H. Ogden, 1994, *Subjects of Analysis*. Lanham, MD: Roman & Littlefield.
12 Heidegger, 1997 [1973], *Phenomenological Interpretation*, cit., p. 164.
13 E. Pound, 1991, *ABC of Reading*. London: Faber & Faber, p. 28.
14 See J.-L. Nancy, 2007 [2002], *Listening*. New York: Fordham University Press, p. 81, n: '*Dicere* is first of all "to show" (e.g. *indicare*); the frequentative *dictare* implies, with repetition and insistance, "saying in a loud voice": as if the sonorous were an intensification of seeing, a placing in tension of present'.
15 R. Barthes, 2007, *Il discorso amoroso. Seminario a l'École Pratique des Hautes Études 1974–1776, seguito da Frammenti di un discorso amoroso (inediti)*. Milano-Udine, Italy: Mimesis, p. 242.

D

DEATH DRIVE. Given that 'drive' is a term which indicates an instinct now taken in the network of language, an instinct thus *distanced* from itself, could the death drive Freud talks about be understood as a rephrasing of what Heidegger meant as the 'being-for-death' as the essence of what is human? But in that sense, it would only be a push to symbolize. And the compulsion to repeat, seemingly blind, would in fact harbour an implicit and vital metaphorizing function.

DEFIANCE. For a healthy development process, the child does not only need to be loved but, as Winnicott writes, 'must also feel real, and if defiance is omitted from the scheme and the child only obeys or identifies, then the child sooner or later complains of lack of feeling real'.[1] Sentences like this nourish my love for psychoanalysis. Short, plain, they make one feel the peaceful experience of the writer, and welcome that of the reader. Surprising in spite of the simplicity of their formulation. They are also a bit mysterious for the particular aura surrounding certain words: *defiance* ... *real* ... like many vortices that may be the origin of something new. It is not easy to define the feeling of being 'real'. If on the one hand one could say that we already knew the value of defiance (just think of the children's pleasure in fighting or the meaning of certain whims), on the other hand it is also true that the way of saying it is new and original. Such a sentence offers relief because, if ever, it lends itself to being used as a happy container for unprocessed proto-emotional elements.

For example, when I read it, it became easier for me to accept why with E. I felt challenged when I told her something that should have been easy to accept and for which I expected quite a bit of gratitude. When it happened the first time, my interpretation was that she wasn't capable of trusting me. I did not realize that *her* way of trusting was precisely the feeling of being able to defy me. Afterwards, I thought that de-identifying oneself was just as necessary as identifying (the etymological meaning of 'to defy' is 'to provoke' or 'to call for battle'/'to challenge').[2] I realized that, on the one hand, an excess of understanding can turn into an intolerable excess of stimuli, and, on the other hand, that, as Winnicott asserts in the same everyday, colloquial but poetic style, 'the infant clings to the thumb and also enjoys separation from it'.[3]

DEPERSONALIZATION. All patients suffer from a certain degree of de-personalization if we understand it as the opposite of the somato-psychic integration condition that is acquired through the process which Winnicott called 'personalization'. That being said, during treatment it is not easy to restart this process because the analyst uses his own defences as well as participating in those of the patient. If I had to say which theoretical-practical principle seems to me to be the most useful in this regard, I would point to the ability to bring everything back to the dream of the session. If he is able to do this, the analyst continually rediscovers that he is the protagonist along with the patient of the spectacle of the analysis and is *forced* to test each time the congruence between rational understanding and affective understanding. The concept of countertransference fulfils the same function, and yet is more limited and therefore less powerful; it operates like a probe but, at least in principle, does not imply that the analyst assumes an equal responsibility for what happens.

DEPRIVATION. A child who is denied the possibility of living affective experiences that can be related to certain unitary elements, that is, of being able to make 'concepts' of them, might suffer from an impairment of the capacity for abstraction. Winnicott expresses something like this when he writes that 'if the mother is lost too long, the transitional object begins to lose value as a symbol'.[4]

DEVIL. This devil of a Winnicott! At the beginning of a review of a book containing the letters sent by Freud to his fiancée, he poses a question: 'Does he [Freud] turn out to be a human human being?'[5] And at the end: 'One could claim that on the evidence of these letters Freud was human'.[6]

DISCOURSE. Barthes's preparatory seminars for his book entitled *A Lover's Discourse: Fragments*[7] are an unparalleled wealth of astonishing suggestions and brilliant insights. It goes without saying that the lover is a figure which can be referred to any patient, no matter what form his suffering has taken. Barthes's book can therefore be considered a true treatise of psychoanalysis.

DON GIOVANNI. In the production of Mozart's Don Giovanni at the Fraschini Theatre in Pavia, in one of the recent seasons, the character of the impetuous knight is dulled by the figure of a boss of our day: a womanizer and cocaine addict. It seems to have been taken entirely form the headlines. The pleasant surprise comes in the end. Instead of the usual sinking into a pit that leads to hell, Don Giovanni gets down and sits among the spectators. Then the lights go out. The split on which the viewer, more or less unconsciously, based his vision throughout the entire opera breaks down. At this point, he cannot help but wonder if, without knowing it, he himself is not dead – if not to life, then at least to vitality. From a scenic gesture, and not an original one either, springs up a disturbing recognition and suddenly Don Giovanni regains his Promethean nobility.

THE DOOR. For some time, the door to my office has been squeaking excruciatingly when opening and closing. It's too heavy and I just cannot solve the issue by myself. I have to wait for a technician to come and fix it. It does not always sound the same. It seems to be affected by the temperature, the weather, and the speed at which I open it and close it. One day, I show a patient out and with surprise and embarrassment I hear the door whistle behind her! Is she thinking what *I* am thinking … ? In retrospect I wonder if this amazing effect does not help me to perceive one aspect of the relationship that I had not considered before. Through a 'sexist' whistle someone less 'civil' or 'polite' enters the scene, an Italian character who might appear in a comic movie by Carlo Verdone. The fact itself had been quite casual (though … why wait so long to fix the door?), but that does not mean that once it has happened it won't be read in all its possible 'field' meanings, conscious and unconscious.

The unexpected and disturbing guest here is seduction, sensuality, the chance of an encounter, not only cold or rational, but one that brings with it the risk of the theatre of analysis, to borrow Freud's expression, being set on fire.

DORA. Freud[8] was embarrassed by the idea that the *Dora* case could be read as a novel because his aim was a naturalistic model of science. Besides the fact that it can be really considered as an extraordinary tale, *Dora* is fascinating because it anticipated the so-called linguistic or rhetorical turn. This formula indicates the postmodern idea that truth cannot be conceived as independent from language, the dwelling place in which the human is shaped, and it does have bases but that these in turn lack them.[9] The only ground on which we can found our truths is that of inter-human agreement. How this agreement is reached remains largely mysterious, we cannot go there and find out the ultimate reasons. To express this notion, Wittgenstein[10] has ingeniously coined the concept of 'language game' (*Sprachspiel*), to which he refers not only specific discursive fields but the whole of culture. In Heidegger,[11] the equivalent is the thematization of the impersonal 'the One /the They' (*das Man*) in *Being and Time*, the analysis of the dark common background from which the subject emerges.

DREAMING. For Bion we dream both night and day. It sounds like the Columbus's Egg. It is easy to understand that all it takes is to let our attention wander off just a little and immediately our mind starts to work the same way it works when it dreams. This is what Freud called the primary process and what Lacan brought back to the play of metonymy and metaphor. However, although this idea might seem bizarre at first, it could have been Descartes who inspired it. No one more than him had focused on the question of the nature of our consciousness and questioned in such a radical way whether, even when we seem to be perceiving a world, we are not just dreaming it. As we know, Descartes admitted that a solution to the problem does not exist, except in a metaphysical order: in his goodness, God could not have confined man to such a solipsistic and desperate situation. The fact remains that the Cartesian argumentation of this point, seen with somewhat half-closed eyes (superimposing the logical impossibility of a definitive distinction on the intuition that there is nothing really to distinguish), at a certain distance, and from a 'secular' perspective where 'deity' is one of the names of O and of the unconscious as the infinity of language, speculatively 'demonstrates' the Bionian assumption.

DREAMS I. Bion:[12] 'Freud [...] took up only the negative attitude, dreams as "concealing" something, not the way in which the *necessary* dream is *constructed*'.

DREAMS II. Shimmering and luminous, enigmatic and transparent, every night dreams make us experience the dizziness of the loss of meaning and as well as of the rebirth of any possible meaning. Only psychoanalysis is able to give back to reason the space of this transcendence.

Works of the dark, like black frames of film, alternating with the exposed ones, dreams reveal the obscurity that is inherent in the light and allow not a simple vision of things. Fragmentary, impalpable, elusive, they appear as absurd theatre performances, one-man-shows for solo spectators.

Dreaming means always being in dialogue with someone. For men it is an activity that cannot be separated from social relations and is not reducible to neurophysiology. Therefore, since thinking is born of the ability to tolerate absence, dreaming is also a conversation with the shadows of a radically alien world. Each time a nocturnal *nekyia*. By dreaming we come into contact with the real and, as Foucault[13] writes, we return to a kind of aquatic communion with the cosmos. How else if not with the body of the mother as our *first home* (Freud)? Do we not experience in dreams the joyful trepidation of a child that looks at himself in her eyes? Are dreams not poems that the mind writes in our sleep to give intimate meaning to this encounter, which then transfigures into existence itself? That is why, as with every happy aesthetic experience, rather than distrust and interpret them as if they concealed unspeakable truths, it is best to let ourselves be interpreted *by* dreams.

DREAMS III. A hotel in Saint-Malô: big, the same one where a few years ago, during a conference, André Green kindly commented on my clinical case. *I'm in the conference room. A French colleague says my name, but I feel paralysed and I cannot answer. Everyone leaves. I wander around the hotel, which looks like a maze. I meet my colleague again, but my torso is naked and I feel embarrassed. I observe the view that you can see from the hotel. A desert-like but fascinating landscape. A mountain shaped like a panettone cake is burning in the distance like a fire. Then there's the waterfall of a river and underneath a beautiful fairytale castle. It reminds me of Mont Saint-Michel.*

DUET. 'Right now, I'm like a cat in heat … ' says Chiara. 'Have you ever heard the female cats when they are in that state? … I always think they keep calling Mauro … Mauro!' Then we talk about something else, and something else again, and finally about nice and ugly names.

I point out that Italian names, especially those derived from Latin, are very beautiful … For example, … Laura … Chiara surprises me and smiles: 'Eh … mAURo … lAURa … mAURo … lAURa … mAURo … !'

Notes

1 D. W. Winnicott, 1989, *Psycho-Analytic Explorations*. Cambridge, MA: Harvard University Press, p. 472.
2 www.etymonline.com/word/defy (Accessed: July 8, 2018).
3 *Ibid.*, p. 436.
4 *Ibid.*, p. 431.
5 *Ibid.*, p. 474.
6 *Ibid.*, p. 477.
7 R. Barthes, 2007, *Il discorso amoroso. Seminario a l'École Pratique des Hautes Études 1974–1976, seguito da Frammenti di un discorso amoroso (inediti)*. Milano-Udine, Italy: Mimesis.
8 S. Freud, 1901, 'Fragment of an analysis of a case of hysteria (Dora)', *The Standard Edition of the Complete Psychological Works of Sigmund Freud (SE)*, vol. 7. London: The Hogarth Press, pp. 1–122.
9 L. Braver, 2014, *Groundless Grounds: A Study of Wittgenstein and Heidegger*. Cambridge, MA: MIT Press.
10 L. Wittgenstein, 2009 [1953], *Philosophical Investigations*. Oxford: Wiley-Blackwell.
11 M. Heidegger, 2010 [1927], *Being and Time*. Albany, NY: SUNY Press.
12 W. R. Bion, 1992, *Cogitations*. London: Karnac Books, p. 33.
13 M. Foucault, 2003 [1994], *Il sogno*. Milano: Raffaello Cortina.

E

ELIOT. After listening to Bion's report at the British Psychoanalytical Society in 1967 entitled 'Negative capability', Winnicott[1] sent him a letter in which instead of attributing the famous sentence about the need to listen to the patient suspending 'memory, desire, understanding, and sense impressions'[2] to Keats, he mentions, perhaps because of a misunderstanding, Eliot's 'version' of the statement, the famous opening passage of *The Waste Land:* 'April is the cruellest month, breeding/Lilacs out of the dead land, mixing/Memory and desire, stirring/Dull roots with spring rain'.[3] In this way, however, Winnicott interprets perfectly Bion's indication because he states that in following it, one is to give up only *voluntary* memory but not the involuntary one. Involuntary memory wakes up suddenly like flowers which appear in spring from the parched winter earth. According to Hinshelwood and Torres the idea is that of a 'generative or regenerative function'[4] of memory.

EMPATHY. Barthes[5] says that this is a word too compromised by sociology to mean 'the consciousness of the social other' and would like it to return 'to a more psychoanalytic sense: empathic coalescence with one's object'. In this definition, which he borrows from Jean Guillaumin, the concept of empathy is very close to that of unison as derived from the Latin *coalescens-entis*, part. pres. of *coalescĕre*, that is to 'join together'.

ENACTMENT. I thought I knew the definition of enactment, but when someone asked me if transformation in hallucinosis was, after all, but another name for enactment, I realized that it was not clear to me. On reflection, the notion of enactment serves to theorize the influence of the analyst's subjectivity and the action component which is also present in the discourse. Still it remains too bound up with the concept of the patient's inevitable misunderstandings due to transference. It is oriented *toward the past* and the search of contents, and less toward the future and the development of the psychic 'container'. Therefore, in the first place, it does not imply the same theoretical reference framework of the analytic field. In the second place, granted that you can accept this perspective, the point is rather *what tools* we have to understand that this is an enactment and what is its meaning.

EURYDICE. Analysts are passionate about meaning. I like to think of their search for meaning as the efforts of Orfeo who moves the Gods with his song in order to bring Eurydice back to life. By this I mean that only looking back we have the impression of being able to make sense of what we have just experienced. And yet, by the mere fact of turning around, meaning (like Eurydice) is dispersed immediately. Could Rilke's verse that invites Orpheus to be 'ever dead in Eurydice'[6] mean that you do not want to force Eurydice out of the shadows, because life and death belong to one another? Being alive means accepting the loss. 'Being dead' in Eurydice reminds us that she is the one who is dead, not the person who has died *in* her (*for* her) and who, instead, nurtures her memory. Eurydice can live in Orpheus, not in herself. Her image, thus, stands for the transience of beauty and of all things.

The myth of Orpheus and Eurydice can then be proposed as an extraordinary figure of the work of the negative to which analysts are constantly dedicated.

EXPIRED OBJECTS. After coming back from her holidays S. tells me her midsummer dream in which I also appeared and seemed to her to be 'in a bad way' (*malandato*). I bitterly muse upon physical problems, the passing years, etc. I also reflect on the meaning of damaged 'object', perhaps because of the summer break and the likely mobilization of aggressive phantasies. But it's only after a couple of hours that the expression comes back to me as in the sense of 'gone away badly' (*male-andato* = *andato-via-male*). What I had seen in a routine perspective came back to me with a more affective quality and with a much richer resonance of meaning. Didn't I say goodbye properly? Did she get angry with me? Had I gone bad (*mal-andato* = *andato a male* = *scaduto*, i.e. 'expired') for her?

Notes

1 N. Torres and R. D. Hinshelwood, 2013, *Bion's Sources: The Shaping of His Paradigms*. London: Routledge.
2 W. R. Bion, 1970, *Attention and Interpretation*. London: Tavistock, p. 43.
3 T. S. Eliot, 1930, *The Waste Land*. New York: Horace Liveright, p. 9.
4 Torres and Hinshelwood, *Bion's Sources*, cit., p. 179.
5 R. Barthes, 2007, *Il discorso amoroso. Seminario a l'École Pratique des Hautes Études 1974–1776, seguito da Frammenti di un discorso amoroso (inediti)*. Milano-Udine, Italy: Mimesis, p. 476.
6 R. M. Rilke, *Sonnets to Orpheus*, translated by M. D. Herter Norton. New York: W.W. Norton & Company, p. 95.

F

FAITH. For Bion, by eschewing memories, desires, understanding and sense impressions, the analyst can approach the field of hallucinosis and 'acts of faith': the only tools with which he can resonate with the 'hallucinations' of his patients and, as a result, learn from experience. Such an attitude is typical of an analyst who 'believes' in the possibility of letting the unconscious do its work. It is obviously not a religious concept, but a term that, for the associations that it arouses, is liable to indicate what can be the ideal state of mind in order to develop the ability for intuition (as opposed to logical/rational thought). For human beings, the meaning lies in a particular point of balance along a continuum Faith↔Fate: between trust which, thanks to the experiences that have nourished our being, we get in the reappearance of the object (meaning, representation) and destiny, as a concept expressing our distress and synonymous with the irrepresentability of death.

We feel the experience as real and authentic as we move between Faith and Fate; when, as Rilke[1] said, we manage to tolerate the terrible, to the point that it seems beautiful, 'the birth of terror'. Each full experience feeds on these basic elements. This applies to life, to art, to analysis. In short, nourishment for the mind is that something which is at the same time captivating and frightening. Every form of meaning, however small, humble and everyday always comes from this *vertigo* (the term is particularly appropriate because it means 'spatial hallucinosis'). But a vertigo that does not make us fall. It is no coincidence that the term has a double meaning, a positive one of surprise and a negative one of disturbance. That is why emotional unison is so important;

because it means the object is here, that it is gone but then it is back (and that will keep coming back). Everything else is secondary, although sophisticated experiences of being at-one, as it were cold/intellectual, can be seen as 'weak' but always useful forms of emotional tuning. The feeling of unison is the aesthetic experience that strengthens the ego.

FASCINATION. I was struggling to understand what I found so fascinating in her. Beauty, of course, but not only. Rather the amused gaze with which she caressed things and people. Sign of acute intelligence and inner harmony, but not only. Perhaps the memory of the loving and kindly ironic look with which the mother's eyes follow the clumsy endeavours of a child? Sometimes, at its peak, that same look in women is mistaken for a sign of a certain empty lightness and as such is *irresistible*. The secret is perhaps that it induces in the other a similar attitude of dreamy and ironic affection: to name it, the most effective way to make him remember the devotion of the object.

FATHERS AND SONS I. On the day of his promotion he receives an email from his old analyst. But there is no text and the subject bar is empty.

FATHER AND SONS II. The father: 'We cannot stay at the seaside much longer, I have to work on Monday'. – The son (six years old): 'That's okay, Dad … you can call in sick!'

FATHERS AND SONS III. 'I saw your book in Freud's house in London!'

FEAR. Antonino Ferro's definition of fear: a cat being barked at (*abbaiato*) by a dog.

FERRANTE. One would have to be able to write like Elena Ferrante. In every line there is a character and an emotion.

FIELD I. In psychoanalysis, it indicates a multidimensional spatiality that is created between patient and analyst at the intersection of the respective bundles of projective identifications. It is a virtual or a fictional space. Attracted in the game of its forces, any object is transformed into an unknown or in a pre-conception and acquires the character of a dream element. The field concept serves to intensify not only abstract or intellectual knowledge but experiential knowledge of the facts of analysis. As a dream, the analytic field is a place where the body is given back to the mind and where the mind can resettle in the body.

FIELD II. For Antonino Ferro, the theory of the analytic field is characterized by two key principles: one ethical, summed up in the Manzonian phrase *omnia munda mundis* (which means that to the pure [men], all things [are] pure); the second theoretical, that everything falls in the dream of the session. The first encourages to not fetishize the rules of the setting, the second to constantly exercise the analytical listening of the unconscious.

FIELD III. Affirming that the field necessarily becomes ill with the patient's illness is a way of reconfirming the theory of transference neurosis, namely that the patient's former infantile neurosis relives in the therapeutic relationship with the analyst. It, therefore, seems contradictory to the very idea of the field, that is, of a space created symmetrically by patient and analyst, and as a psychoanalytic treatment model in which the foreground is the current emotional experience as seen through the prism of the concept of the session as a dream. In fact there is no contradiction, because even knowing their weight, in the interest of a more effective cure practice you decide tactically to put aside the historical determinants of mental suffering which are the object of the cure. More precisely, the history and the background of understanding that it provides are not cancelled, but are captured at a metanarrative level starting from the vertex of emotional transformations in the analytic field.

THE FITS. A poetic, beautiful and original film (72nd Venice Film Festival, College Section). Tony (Royalty Hightower) is an 11-year-old girl who does boxing in a Cincinnati gym where she goes with her older brother. The hobby reflects her shut-off and tormented personality. At one point, however, dragged along by Beezy, her cheerful and charming younger friend, she becomes fascinated by a group of colourful cheerleaders (the Lionesses) who are practising for a dance contest in the adjoining room. Seeing how Toni manages to gradually integrate, first awkwardly and then more harmoniously, her deadly boxing blows into dance movements, literally opens to the dream about a series of essential things in life, but that's why I would like to leave them unsaid, at least here. It would be interesting to read the film in a psychoanalytic perspective, but what strikes me is quite the opposite:

how *The Fits*[2] is able to interpret the 'choreographic' nature of the analytic relationship.

FLYING DUTCHMAN. The flying Dutchman in Wagner's opera can 'die', or, experience a new bond and live in an authentic way, only when he finds a woman who has been faithful to him until death, that is who restores a maternal presence inside of him which would be a source of faith. We could see their death in the final scene of the opera as an allegory of the acceptance of the transience of things, a variation of the Leopardian theme of 'sweet shipwreck' or of the 'slow death' in the arms of his beloved in one of D'Annunzio's[3] most extraordinary poems. A slow death which is actually an authentic living. Instead, not to accept the terrible means to live being neither dead nor alive.

FOG I. (E. at the door, leaving the office) 'It's very foggy out there today!'

FOG II. One book can change your life. Ever since I read the praise for fog composed by Sergio Vitale[4] in his *Si prega di chiudere gli occhi: Esercizi di cecità volontaria* [*Close Your Eyes: Voluntary Blindness Exercises*], nothing in Pavia was the same: 'By the subtle collapse of identity which it provokes in the heart of reality, the gaze finally finds its original, primordial state from back when "seeing" meant merely "perceiving", always an instant before any thought or language'. Vitale goes on to describe it as the unformed 'original womb, within which all things are held together, emerging and sinking into the foam of being, ignoring any pre-established hierarchy, insensitive to every call of expectation'.

FREUD. Freud thinks within a positivist framework and looks mainly at the *nature* of instincts about to become drives. This is why he defines them as something between the somatic and the psychic (obviously a human psychic). Less conditioned by biology, Bion instead starts from *culture* and uses emotion to put the relationship, the birth of conscience, back at the centre of the analytical work and theory; which is like saying what underpins it: access to language. Both aim to explain the essence of human being, but choose different perspectives leading to different clinical practices.

FULL STOP. In the text from a session the patient discussed, A. is sometimes referred to as 'A.' but sometimes as 'Alessandra', 'the patient', or even simply 'A' (no full stop). It also happens that, in reading the report, my colleague completes the name by transforming it from 'A' or 'A.' to 'Alessandra' and by that noticing that in the group work the patient is being progressively 'humanized'. In the story of her life, it is noted that somehow at eleven years of age, at the threshold of puberty, A. has 'put a full stop' to her emotional growth, but not to the intellectual one. 'Here's the "full stop"', someone suggested, meaning, the interruption of development. In one passage of a dialogue A. ends her sentence with a pause and an ellipsis ('Yes. That's right, when he does this I burst into uncontrollable rage and then it's better if I mark some borders …'). The analyst replies with reference to the need to build dams and then, immediately afterwards, she lingers on her own reveries. She thinks of 'the flooding of the Tigris and Euphrates in …..' (five dots), and says that 'if the water retreated, it left the ground more fertile, if it did not withdraw, it formed a swamp making the soil no longer cultivable'. *Meso*potamia as an intermediate area of analysis and emotional flooding thus finds an effective representation together with the awareness of their inevitability and utility, *provided that they then retreat.* Regarding the ongoing dialogue, we wondered if it could indicate, as it were in real time, Alessandra's emotional attitude, but also her 'usual' way of reacting to things: with a sudden braking and raising of ramparts or retreating into mental shelters. Obviously, the same indication could apply to the analyst. Likewise, in the text the husband is marked as 'M.' or 'Matteo' or 'the husband'. At the beginning of the text A. comes across as a 'nun', angelic, heavenly: three dots or a full stop for libido! Her desires are like the books she loved, but which she locked away in a library which is difficult to access because she is allergic to dust.

FUNCTION. It cannot be said that Kant's influence on Bion has been sufficiently recognized. Kant is the author in which the Copernican revolution of transcendental schematism (for the subject, knowing means to modify oneself) intersects the theory of the sublime, which can be considered a true pre-psychoanalytic doctrine of subjectivation. For instance, the role played by the concept of 'function' in Kant is well known. If it is not taken into account, one does not immediately grasp the meaning of Bion's reformulation of the concept of the unconscious as a 'psychoanalytic function of personality'. The formula means that the unconscious, which should be written in a verbal form, as 'unconsciousing' since it is a set of processes, is a 'spontaneous' but not innate function of the psyche that 'treats' the sensory and emotional raw data in order to give them meaning. The adjective 'psychoanalytic' simply reminds us that it is a psychoanalytic theory. The value of Bion's theorization is to shape a theory and practice of psychoanalysis (the famous Freudian *Junktim*) that goes beyond the limits of Kant's discourse already pointed out by Hegel and Heidegger. For example, not having had the courage to trace back the foundation of being to the dark root of a sociality that is not thematizable and therefore being pulled back while facing this task that has become less and less eludible over time.

FUTURE PSYCHOANALYSIS. Berlin 2014, a conference called 'Psychoanalysis 2025'. Not a lot of new ideas, some of them 'implied': a serious one, holding the conference at a University of Psychoanalysis; another semi-serious one: choosing to put the speakers up in a hotel called *Abion* ('a-Bion', I could not help but translate: an ambiguous indication of the new paradigms of psychoanalysis directed towards Bion [in Italian, the preposition 'a' indicates movement to a place], but also alpha privative). I still got something out of it. Realizing the annoying insistence in defining psychoanalysis not by an extremely sophisticated practice of listening to the unconscious and the systematic exercise of doubt but by the extrinsic parameters of the the number of sessions, it never seemed to me clearer that this is how you end up in a dead-end street and that the only possible way out is to develop new ideas. Moreover, those which could be considered as alternatives to obsolete models are not all that new and have been in circulation for some time. No new answers to old questions that turned out not to be heuristic anymore, but simple answers to new questions.

Notes

1 R. M. Rilke, 1931 [1923], *Duineser Elegien: Elegies from the Castle of Duino*, translated by V. & E. Sackville West. London: Hogarth Press, p. 4.
2 A. R. Holmer (director), *The Fits*, USA, 2015.
3 G. D'Annunzio, 1939, 'Sopra un "Erotik" di Edvard Grieg', in: *L'orto e la prora*. Roma: La Fondazione, 'Il Vittoriale degli Italiani', p. 37.
4 S. Vitale, 2007, *Si prega di chiudere gli occhi. Esercizi di cecità volontaria.* Firenze: Clinamen, pp. 12–13.

G

GRID. In Bion, both a periodic table of the psychic elements and a sort of Cartesian diagram to study the 'subatomic physics' of the development of thought.

GROUP. Bion sees the two-person session in analogy to those of the leaderless group designed to select army officers, and of group psychotherapy sessions at the hospital in Northfield during World War II. The technique is the same: the analyst refuses to lead the patient and waits for emotional tension lines to show. By adapting the concepts to the dual situation, from a careful re-reading of *Experiences in Groups*,[1] one could draw up a manual of psychoanalysis. For example, the characters of the dialogue would be the indexes of the basic assumptions active in the analytical field.

In this regard, I do not think that the influence on Bion's thought of John Rickman, his first analyst and later collaborator and co-author, has been sufficiently recognized. However, looking at their correspondence one can get a good idea of it.[2]

Notes

1 W. R. Bion, 1998 [1961], *Experiences in Groups and Other Papers*. London: Routledge.

2 G. Civitarese, 2011, 'Towards an ethics of responsibility', *International Forum Psychoanalysis*, 20:108–112.

H

HALLUCINOSIS. Hallucinosis is a condition in which a person maintains a lucid consciousness while still experiencing hallucinations. In psychiatry, the possible causes are organic or pharmacological. Imported into psychoanalysis, the term indicates not true hallucinations, but invisible, negative hallucinations. The subject expels their mental content into the outer world, forming a sort of film that reassures and protects them from the threat posed by all that is alien to them.

The model of hallucinosis is the dream, which closes the sensory channels and creatively reworks elements of the interior landscape to paint the emotions. The hallucinosis is thus, analogously to the dream, a *via regia* to this landscape. If understood as co-created, even the hallucinosis of the analyst will never be only *his*, but will express the qualities of the unconscious emotional field shared by the couple. For the analyst, then, hallucinosis becomes a probe with which to explore the analytic field.

One could say that in the state of waking we are always dreaming a dream which we are not aware of and that the aim of interpretation is to awaken from this unknowingness and to make a dream into a real dream. What's peculiar to hallucinosis is that it is of a quantitative and not of a qualitative nature, so much so that hallucinosis is sometimes called a psychosis of daily life. Pathological hallucinosis, on the other hand, is the sign of a lack of balance. Finally, hallucinosis, as an analyst's tool to maximize receptivity, is a kind of self-induced illness for therapeutic purposes, and consists in putting to one side memories, desires, and theories as much as it's possible. In the end it is just a strict application of a principle known in phenomenology as transcendental reduction, except for the fact that, like a dream during the night, it cannot be produced at will; we can only lay the groundwork for it to appear.

HANDS. She gave the impression, from what I could see from behind the couch, to talk more with her hands than with her voice. What did her hands say? They spoke of desire and anguish. To understand it I was aided by two lines from *Salomé* by Oscar Wilde, which I had reread recently, after seeing Al Pacino's[1] film with Jessica Chastain as the bloodthirsty princess, and which I associated with the scene: 'The Princess has hidden her face behind her fan! Her little white hands are fluttering like doves that fly to their dovecots. They are like white butterflies. They are just like white butterflies.'[2] What a scary movie!

HISTORY AND INTERSUBJECTIVITY. Husserl[3] defines history as 'from the start nothing other than the vital movement of the coexistence [*Miteinander*] and the interweaving [*Ineinander*] of original formations and sedimentations of meaning'. In the original the terms *Miteinander* and *Ineinander* better render the double level of interpersonal and intersubjective interaction underpinning the existence of the *animal rationalis*. Compared to the first (the interpersonal relationship), which expresses the *meaning* exchanged between two subjects, the second (the intersubjective relationship) rather takes into account commerce in *sense* which always precedes it and then always accompanies it, and which occurs on a pre-categorical level. One could say that it is not history that makes the subject but intersubjectivity that inaugurates history. Any historical fact, continues Husserl, has its necessary and 'inner structure of meaning', which is mostly unexamined:

> All [merely] factual history remains incomprehensible because, always merely drawing its conclusions naïvely and straightforwardly from facts, it never makes thematic the general ground of meaning upon which all such conclusions rest, has never investigated the immense structural a priori which is proper to it.[4]

One might wonder if it is not by answering a similar objection, transposed into its field, that psychoanalysis has come to give priority to the terrain of *sense* over that of *meaning*; where sense is identifiable with affection and in general with the aesthetic dimension of the therapeutic relationship, in which the facts of analysis are rooted.

HOLOPHRASIS. The analysand's discourse is essentially holophrastic. It is equivalent to those single words or interjections pronounced by the infant that have the value of an entire speech. Moreover, what holophrasis expresses is a request for love. Just like the lover's *I-love-you* is nothing but a repeated *tell-me-you-love-me* in the palimpsest of language. This is an appeal addressed to the other to transform according to one's own desire. Now, what is interesting in this concept is, on the one hand, the reference to the impotent state of the infant and, on the other, the image of the total immersion of the subject, as Julia Kristeva[5] observes, in motor activity or in a gestural language.

HUMAN. I present a clinical case at the B*, a traditional stronghold of ego psychology. Afterwards a distinguished fellow of the Institute says, reassured, that my style of work resonated with him very well. I thought that maybe he had been expecting to see green antennae popping out of my head as if I were a Martian.

The scene is repeated at the Tavistock Clinic in London a few months later although with reversed parts, because here in the foreground is the fear of orthodoxy. During the coffee break, one of the participants of the seminar on dreams approaches shyly and says: 'You know, I'm a "transpersonal" [?]. This morning, knowing that there would be a psychoanalyst here, I said, "My God … no … a psychoanalyst!" Then, when you started talking … Well … I thought … he seems human … !'

HYPERTENSION. During an analysis, a patient gets high blood pressure and tells the analyst about it. How do I listen to what he's saying? It depends on the role we have. If I were his cardiologist, I would invite him to make a series of diagnostic tests, I would suggest a diet, I would recommend some lifehygiene measures and I'd prescribe him medication. As an analyst I could think that if a patient has started suffering from hypertension, it could be because of an excess of stimuli which he cannot 'digest', and which is therefore a source of stress. I could relate the symptom to unconscious aspects of his behaviour in affective relationships. For example, hypothesizing that there is a link with a chronically suppressed anger which is activated in certain oedipal situations, inside and outside the analysis. This would help to have a new perspective on things and maybe change his attitude.

But there is also another possibility: to consider *hyper*tension as a character in the fictional dialogue of analysis to express something that concerns the unconscious communication in the here and now. I could try to develop the narration of this character. The aim would be to ensure that the patient is equipped with the best tools to interpret his reality and thus to give meaning to certain situations with no need for the hypertension-character to enter the scene (a kind of a Hulk always on the verge of exploding).

Which of the procedures described is the most effective? In my opinion, the one with which you can see better what is happening in the present on the unconscious level of communication. Of course, nothing prevents the analyst from talking about the connection between office conflicts and hypertension as long as he knows that he is also talking about something that is happening in the consulting room. In this way, he uses an integrated, binocular vision and does not risk separating the present emotions by encapsulating them in alleged realities outside of the analysis or in transference manifestations understood as one-way misunderstandings.

HYPOCHONDRIA. The hypochondriac suffers from sense, not from meaning. The crisis of meaning (what gives strength and direction to the subject) is always a crisis of affectivity. Hence the ruthless scrutiny of the body, because suddenly the 'written' body becomes indecipherable. The fact is that one's own body (sensible, readable, focused) is born from the identification with the object. By 'fetishsizing' an organ, the hypochondriac rummages through his own flesh, not in his own body, but in the body of the object. Likewise, a lover scrutinizes the face of a beloved person to find out why they are no longer wanted.

In the extreme case, Barthes[6] suggests, this scholarly perspective can 'move from *in vivo* to *in vitro*, that is, to make the body of the other inert, and to desire to possess this inertia. Not sadism, since victims of sadism should cooperate and even rejoice, but rather a necrophilic drive.' Would the necrophile passion, as seen in some serial killer films, such as *The Cell*,[7] be then the vicious and hyperbolic stage of hypochondrial anxiety?

Notes

1 A. Pacino (director), *Wilde Salomé*, USA, 2011.
2 O. Wilde, 1922 [1891], *Salome*. Girad, KA: Haldeman-Julius, p. 9.
3 E. Husserl, 1989 [1939], 'The origin of geometry', in: J. Derrida, ed., *Edmund Husserl's Origin of Geometry: An Introduction*. Lincoln, NE; London: University of Nebraska Press, p. 174.
4 *Ibid.*
5 J. Kristeva, 1984 [1974]. *Revolution in Poetic Language*. New York: Columbia University Press, p. 267.
6 R. Barthes, 2007, *Il discorso amoroso. Seminario a l'École Pratique des Hautes Études 1974–1776, seguito da Frammenti di un discorso amoroso (inediti)*. Milano-Udine, Italy: Mimesis, p. 472.
7 T. Singh (director), *The Cell*, USA, 2000. See also the chapter on this film in: G. Civitarese, 2018 [2013], *The Necessary Dream: New Theories and Techniques of Interpretation in Psychoanalysis*. London: Routledge.

I

IDEA. Winnicott[1] writes: 'This contact of the nipple with the baby's mouth gives the baby ideas! – "perhaps there is something there outside the mouth worth going for"'. What intrigues me in this sentence is the word 'idea'. We cannot think of it as an idea in the proper sense, that is, an idea had by someone who can think his thoughts. It has to be a rather special, rudimentary idea, a 'bodily idea'. Likewise, Bion speaks of the 'conception' that arises from the encounter of a pre-conception with a realization. Unlike the term 'concept', 'conception' has more to do with an idea of process and is better suited to indicate a concept that is more of a pre-reflective order – as a kind of dance in which you are engaged with the other – than a psychic content of the representational type.

IN SIMPLE TERMS. It is true that at times what the patient needs the most is a 'little bath of words', a happy expression of Didier Anzieu. But for the most part the analyst should not use too many words. Using few, simple words, expresses in itself an ethics of hospitality, creates a concave and welcoming space for the other. The power of silence and of the negative is thus placed at the service of a maieutic of form. Answering questions with silence, sometimes even with a silence that can be found *in* words, also serves to leave the unconscious time to do its job.

INFINITE. In the poem 'The Infinite' Leopardi systematically uses the same figure of speech which Longinus recommended in his treatise to authors in order to obtain the sublime: hyperbaton (or anastrophe). Every line has the words in a reversed order in such a way that at first it is difficult to grasp the meaning. It therefore 'collapses' threateningly on the reader because meaning is suspended and could be terrible (any absence of meaning is). It is only in its second part that the sentence stretches out and restores the space that in the perspectival view of things we identify with rationality.[2] Thanks to the reiteration of this expressive pattern, in each verse the drama with a happy ending is told of extricating oneself from the suffocating embrace of the object made again *ab-ject* (i.e. placed at a safe distance). The same movement is also achieved in terms of content because with its mysterious nature, the allegory ('the last horizon') precedes the explanation of the allegorized ('the dead seasons'). It brings to mind Lacan's[3] observation in seminar X about the danger posed not so much by the absence of the object but by its immanence.

INSTANCE. Instance derives from the Latin word *instantia*, which comes from *instare* or 'to insist', 'to urge', 'to be above' and has several meanings. From 'need' or 'necessity' to a request addressed to an authority, and finally an organization or institution endowed with the power of decision-making. The ego-as-instance consists in *insisting* on questioning the object, on challenging the sphinx. Sometimes, as in Kafka's 'A Message from the Emperor', no response is received. As it turns out, the response was in waiting, in desire.

INTERCOM. A. rings the doorbell. I open. I hear it ringing again. I press the button again to open the main door. Shortly after, the patient is on the threshold of the study and, panting after climbing the stairs, says to me: 'Did I ring twice?!' 'Yes, but I already opened after the first time', I reply. Once on the couch A. resumes: 'You did not expect me today!' And me: 'Of course I did!' We reconstruct what must have happened. In fact, I had the impression that the new next door neighbour answered the intercom by mistake. A. confirms this and adds that, indeed, the question 'Who is it?' to which she did not answer, was asked in a voice that was 'dull, different from yours and *a bit hostile* … kind of *wolfish*'. That's why she did not come in and rang a second time. The 'hallucination' of the neighbour, who attributed the ringing to his doorbell, and which for a little while had been somehow also ours, once transformed into a hallucinosis, that is, into a hallucination we are now aware of, gives us the possibility of thinking of another 'neighbour' – I for her and she for me – unexpected and fierce, to some animalistic ferocity that might concern us. 'The walls of these houses are so thin', she says to me. Had she not, by the hostility in my voice, been able to conclude that I was not expecting her today?

INTERMEDIARITY. Psychoanalysis belongs to the intermediate world. This essential truth is expressed in various concepts: transference (Freud), transitional space (Winnicott), 'something between' (Bion), the intersubjective analytic third (Ogden), the analytic field (Ferro).

INTERPERSONALISM I. B*, November 2015. A. presents a case where there is no trace of any listening oriented to guess the unconscious sense of communication, as should be the norm. Afterwards, in a nice French restaurant, a witty colleague, quoting Gertrud Stein, remarks: '*There was no there there*'.

INTERPERSONALISM II. At the heart of every model of psychoanalysis there is a search for truth and the belief that truth is what nourishes the mind – it could not be any other way, if by truth we mean the product of inter-human consensuality. All of them make then the next step and try to get to know this truth through experience lived with the patient in the here and now of the session. Immediacy would be a guarantee. However, this factor is theorized with very different nuances in the various cases that can yield the interpretation of transference (Freud's model), of unconscious phantasies (Kleinian model), of the characters of the session (field model) or of enactments (interpersonal model). In each of these models, the unconscious is assigned a variable weight. Curiously enough, approaches which are to a certain extent similar, such as the field and interpersonal models, are on opposing poles with respect to this parameter. In fact, relational models are based on a phenomenological reduction that is similar to that of the field, but in a much more partial manner and above all by preserving a traditional notion of subject and of unconscious. Not of the unconscious, as Bion outlines it, seen as the psychoanalytic function of the personality, but the repressed unconscious of classical theory. For Bion, analysis means 'unconsciousing', i.e. making unconscious what is conscious or starting a process of learning from experience that goes to enrich the un/conscious apparatus for symbolization of the subject. On the contrary, as Henri Smith says: 'The more "empirical" North American approaches would, I believe, be viewed by many European analysts, and by some North Americans as well, as distractions from the task of analysing unconscious fantasy and unconscious defenses'.[4] Rachael Blass,[5] quoting Smith, comments:

> The second form of 'here and now' that has become dominant in psychoanalysis may be referred to as an interpersonal approach. Here, in the effort to stay with what is most immediate, the analytic focus shifts to the actual relationship between the patient and the analyst – what is being experienced and what may be understood – but the unconscious depths are downplayed [...] What become less significant are the unconscious determinants of the relationship and the fact that they are being *relived* in the present relationship.

And more:[6] 'As we have seen, these other "here and now" approaches seek immediacy and wish to avoid intellectualization, but in so doing do not tie between immediacy and depth, between experience and unconscious truth'. Well said!

INTERPRETATION I. The best definition of interpretation I ever came across was given by Heidegger in the preface to his book on the poetry of Hölderlin. He writes that interpretation should be like snow falling on a bell and then disappearing without a trace. It is obvious, we could say, that no one will ever forget the spectacle of snowflakes dancing in the air and of the white, snow-covered ground. Heidegger concludes: 'The last, but also the most difficult step of every interpretation, consists in its disappearing'.[7]

INTERPRETATION II. Speaking of the *style* of interpretation, in tune with that of the above-mentioned German philosopher is the page in Calvino's[8] *Invisible Cities* about Marozia. There's the idea that, when you least expect it, at every turn of the road, it looks like a different city. And then the sight immediately disappears. Spaces, heights and dimensions change continuously. It is not known how and why. Perhaps it is a question of being able to look in a certain way or say special words. Perhaps it is a question of pace. What is essential, however, is that everything should happen as it happens by chance, without intention.The analytical conversation also has the erratic tendency of a hypertext[9] or of a talking-as-dreaming.[10] It seems to me that what emerges here is an idea of interpretation as an 'adventure'. There is the sense of wandering that can make one tumble down suddenly (πίπτω)[11] and face an unexpected misfortune, but also of an event that, though with difficulty, ends well, somewhat undecided between disaster and dissolution.

INTERPRETATION III. In interpreting, the analyst should adapt one poetic principle set out by film director Mikael Haneke: enter in the scene as late as possible and leave it as soon as possible. The same applies to the Bressonian essentiality which characterizes his style.

INTERPRETATION IV. The analyst should not interpret but have a 'conversation' with the patient in a way that makes them both more *humane*. As an exercise to practice talking in a simple and real way, it helps a lot to imagine saying the same thing at a bar to a close friend. Any annoying traces of jargon are shaken off from the sentences and they are immediately brought back to life.

INTERPRETATION V. In Winnicott[12] we find a surprising reversal of the usual way of understanding interpretation. It is when the analyst is silent that he understands what is happening and not when he speaks:

> one of the purposes of interpreting is to establish the limits of the analyst's understanding. The basis for not interpreting and in fact not making any sound at all is the theoretical assumption that the analyst really does know what is going on.

INTERSPACE. At the 14th edition of the Venice Bienniale of Architecture (2014), Estonia presented an installation called *Interspace*. A projection system intercepted the movements of the visitors and translated them into bright lines on a floor divided into many regular frames. I was pleasantly surprised to find that when suddenly children started running, the lines they drew were curved and colourful and no longer black and geometrical! The children's trajectories suggested play, while those of adults – rational thinking. However, in the happiest moments of analysis, one plays also with adults. By not worrying about generating meanings, there remains only one – but maybe the most important one of all – meaning without meaning, that of *dance*. A dance of colourful words. As Pound wrote, in order to be effective, poetry should be music and music – dance.

INTERSUBJECTIVE. Often mistaken for what refers to the interaction between two separate entities rather than the intermediate area or space between them, *in-between*. In fact there are psychic elements which cannot develop exclusively in one's head, without the participation of the other (and of the *O*ther, accordingly to Lacanian slang), but can only be born, as is the case of language, *among* individuals. The term therefore refers to the subject's *social* constitution, but understood in Husserl's and Merleau-Ponty's sense of *Ineinandersein*;[13] that is to say, of the *being in each other* – an interconnection/binding which is initially concrete/sensorial, and only later on is followed by ideas – that constitues us as human beings.

IPHONE I. R. tells me about the torment from which he's been suffering for a long time because he cannot decide whether to live with A. or B. From the coat rack at the entrance to the office comes the sound of his mobile phone ringtone: a carefree whistling, airy and slightly ironic.

IPHONE II. A completely silent session. At the door, before leaving, A. unplugs the cell phone that had been charging at the electrical outlet near the *Ficus benjamina* plant, checks the power level of the appliance and exclaims: 'Still, at least something got done!'

ISTANBUL. November 6, 2015, a French analyst: 'Je ne dis pas que la psychanalyse française soit meilleure que la vôtre!'

Notes

1 D. W. Winncott, 1978 [1964, 1957], *The Child, the Family and the Outside World*. Harmondsworth: Penguin Books, p. 46.

2 See S. Vitale, 2015, *Il paesaggio e il suo rovescio. Distanza e proiezione nel luogo dell'altro*. Firenze: Clinamen.

3 J. Lacan, 2014 [2004], *Anxiety: The Seminar of Jacques Lacan, Book X*. Cambridge: Polity Press.

4 H. F. Smith, 2003, 'Analysis of transference: A North American perspective', *International Journal of Psychoanalysis*, 84:1017–1041, p. 1028.

5 R. B. Blass, 2011, 'On the immediacy of unconscious truth: Understanding Betty Joseph's "here and now" through comparison with alternative views of it outside of and within Kleinian thinking', *International Journal of Psychoanalysis*, 92:1137–1157, p. 1141.

6 *Ibid.*, p. 1154.

7 M. Heidegger, 2000, *Elucidations of Hölderlin's Poetry*. New York: Humanity Books, p. 22.
8 I. Calvino, 1974, *Invisible Cities*. New York: Houghton Mifflin Harcourt.
9 G. Civitarese, 2008, *The Intimate Room: Theory and Technique of the Analytic Field*. London: Routledge.
10 T. H. Ogden, 2008, *Rediscovering Psychoanalysis: Thinking and Dreaming, Learning and Forgetting*. London: Routledge.
11 www.etimo.it/?term=peripezia&find=Cerca (Accessed: March 8, 2016).
12 D. W. Winnicott, 1989, *Psycho-Analytic Explorations*. Cambridge, MA: Harvard University Press, p. 85.
13 See D. Morton, 2016, '*Ineinandersein* and *L'interlacs*: The constitution of the social world or "we-world" in E. Husserl and M. Merleau-Ponty', in: T. Szanto and D. Morton, eds., *Phenomenology of Sociality: Discovering the 'We'*. London: Routledge, p. 108.

J

JEALOUSY. R. seems to suffer not so much because she was cheated on but because with betrayal an unrivalled potential of beauty has been destroyed. The divine face of the object has suddenly turned into the sneer of a monster.

The violence that can result from pathological jealousy does not mainly derive from a feeling of exclusion of an oedipal nature. Nor can the moving reference to lost beauty be read according to the dynamics of a grieving process. On the contrary, in the good form by now destroyed, the true Self which had had to be hidden and remained secret because rejected by the object in the primary relation and therefore reduced to monstrosity, returns to despair. The false Self that defended it was finally unmasked and dismantled the defence that it represented for the subject.

JOYCE?!. The patient in the case presented for supervision had suffered all the traumas that could be suffered in childhood due to a great neglect on the part of the mother. A colleague, a militant feminist, comes up with an incomprehensible interpretation by drawing a comparison to the relationship between Dedalus and Bloom in Joyce's masterpiece. I gently manifest some cautious scepticism. My colleague goes into a tantrum. 'Always the mothers, always the mothers!', she growls. 'The other day two "radicalized" Islamists killed fifteen people in Texas … and it is always the mother's fault!'

Not being an Islamist, or even a Catholic for that matter, and least of all a radicalized one … what in the bloody hell have I done to her?!, I wonder. It's amazing how in a matter of seconds violent emotions can be ignited within a group, and usually by its most fragile participants; those emotions that Bion called basic assumptions.

On that occasion, I managed to keep calm and make good use of the accident: *now that we had the patient's mother, we no longer had to imagine her!* Here is what according to Bion is meant by transformation in O as opposed to transformation in K, that is, getting to know through experience and not just abstractly.

K

KAFKA. At the exhibition called 'La grande madre' [*The Big Mother*][1] at the Palazzo Reale in Milan, among the most interesting works was the reconstruction of the torture machine invented by Kafka in the story entitled *In the Penal Colony*. Not only was the sentence engraved in blood on one's skin, but after the etching was finished, you could not even read it. The words were in fact hidden by graphic ornaments of the text.

KLEIN. Winnicott: 'if Melanie Klein had not existed we would have had to have invented her'.[2] One of my patients: 'Rubbish! … with Freud there is at least hope but with Klein you're screwed!'

Notes

1 M. Gioni, 2015, 'La grande madre'. Milano: Skira.

2 D. W. Winnicott, 1989, *Psycho-Analytic Explorations*. Cambridge, MA: Harvard University Press, p. 467.

L

LANGUAGE OF EFFECTIVENESS. This is how F. describes it to me while putting together an acclamation speech for a colleague: 'He writes effective sentences … it seems that they have nothing to do with anything and yet they create powerful connections …'.

LAST SUMMER. Leonardo Seràgnoli's[1] film picks up its central theme from Bertolucci's *The Last Emperor*: the lacerating pain of a child being separated from the mother. A luxurious yacht off the coast of Otranto. Four crewmembers, a six-year-old boy named Ken and his young Japanese mother together for the last four days before a separation that will last until the boy's coming of age, as dictated by the conditions of the divorce settlement. During their short holiday, the mother regains the affection of the child, who initially rejects her. From the beginning she shows signs of mental instability and the crew members are very tense. The viewer expects something tragic to happen at any moment. But nothing happens. In the last beautiful scene, the mother leaves after giving the baby a cloth mask which she has made herself. The mask is oriental, colourful, and grotesque, a mask of an old man, perhaps a demon. The child, by now left alone, puts it on, wanders around the ship's deck, and then looks at us, as if we have become the eyes of his mother. The narrative solution is brilliant. *Seemingly* nothing happens, but in fact something dramatic, perhaps definitive, takes place in Ken's soul. Suddenly his face has become old, deformed, perhaps evil. In a flash, his life closed off in the circle of an invisible prison.

LEARNING FROM EXPERIENCE. May 2012, a clinical supervision with the Kleinian group in B*. There is a theological dispute with a follower of Lacan. November 2015, another supervision for the same group. The same follower starts insinuating: 'But what do you mean by "real"? Is it the same as Lacan's "real"?!' 'For goodness sake, NOOO – I answer – I don't really know much about Lacan!!' Reassured, she smiles at me. When the meeting was finished, a participant in the group says that he admires my ability to learn from experience.

LEOPARDI. In Mario Martone's film *Leopardi*[2] some of the most poetic moments are those in which the historical coherence of the setting is violated by a pop soundtrack. However, the metaleptic short circuit between the worlds resonates with Leopardi's ingenious ability to capture temporality, to make the past more distant and vice versa – in projecting the present in the past.

LICHTENBERG. After having asked me right after the summer to temporarily reduce the number of our sessions from three to one, M. tells me that for a couple of weeks it might prove difficult for her to come to that one session because she has to take her children to preschool. I immediately think of the Lichtenberg's knife, mentioned by Freud[3] when talking about Jung: a bladeless knife with no handle. In other words: there is no analysis left; or: how to make the object magically disappear. However, the image of the knife is surprising. I wonder if what is happening should not serve to introduce a certain violence into the analysis. But, whose knife? we could ask.

One could think that for some reason M. feels threatened and that is why – and it is understandable – he runs away. In turn, I feel attacked and I realize that I often get bored with him and that lately I have become quite cold towards him. Nor is the context of Freud's quote alien to the reverie, which is that of bitterness and of his disappointment with Jung, his chosen son.

Lichtenberg's knife is, thus, a way of evoking *nothingness* but leaving a trace of its disappearance. Ultimately as in the *fort/da* game, playing with the absence or, even better, perpetuating the alternation of appearance and disappearance from which the capacity to represent is born. Hit by strong emotions because of my upcoming 'dismissal' by M., I unconsciously try to reconstruct a possible meaning and, thus, to keep a little control over things. And if it is true that the reverie, like the dream, puts us directly in touch with thoughts of the waking dream, then I can draw a more precise map of the emotions that switch on in the analytical field and, therefore, try to transform them.

LITMUS TEST. What would be the litmus test to see if you are not talking to the patient in an artificial way or in jargon? Imagine asking someone to guess what 'narrative genre' the piece of dialogue belongs to. If they answer correctly that is the voice of an analyst, you are on the wrong track.

LOST AND FOUND.

patients forget small items:
a blue scarf
a guitar pick
wait, that's a pick … a patient who plays the guitar! – she says
a black purse with white polka dots for pencils and small stationary
but is that purse yours? – she asks ironically and a little astonished
objects never requested back
a funny umbrella with ducks above it
in the end I adopted them
but they are still there to reclaim their rightful owner
I pitifully put them away

LOVE. About *Gradiva*, Barthes[4] writes: 'Freud assimilates here, in a certain way, loving cure and psychoanalytic cure: […] we must not underestimate the curative power of love in delusion'. And also:

> The issue at stake in the Gradivian technique: […] to *recognize* the subject in love as a subject, that is, to prove to him his own existence, his own value, and to want to teach him something about himself. This recognition must be *indirect*.[5]

Prior to Searles, Loewald, and Ogden, it was considered taboo to speak frankly about love in analysis (*where, for that matter, we never talk about anything else*) because it immediately brought to mind the fire at the theatre, the image used by Freud to evoke the ruinous transgression of the rules of the analytic frame.

To say that in analysis what cures is a sort of *indirect* love is neither a false statement nor an exaggeration. Bion writes that the mother loves her child with her 'capacity for reverie'. The most beautiful description of love in analysis that I know is found in Ogden's[6] essay, 'Reading Harold Searles', which appeared in his book *Rediscovering Psychoanalysis*. Commenting on Searles's

'Oedipal love in counter transference', Ogden argues that in order to successfully analyse oedipal love, the analyst must fall in love with the patient, recognizing that his desires can never be realized and will always remain in the sphere of sentiment.[7] Chetrit-Vatine[8] speaks of analysis as a situation of mutual seduction, which naturally, on the analyst's part, must remain 'ethical'. Kristeva[9] also sees a 'new kind of love story' in the transference; and, in the request for therapy, a lack of love which can only be filled by experiencing the transference bond: 'complaints, symptoms, or fantasies are discourses of love directed to an impossible other – always unsatisfactory, transitory, incapable of meeting my wants and desires'. Besides, according to Jean Laplanche, the child's psychic birth is founded upon the mother's primary seduction.

Notes

1 L. G. Seràgnoli (director), *Last Summer*, Italia, 2014.
2 M. Martone (director), *Leopardi*, Italia, 2014.
3 S. Freud, 1916, 'The history of the psychoanalytic movement', *Psychoanalytic Review*, 3:406–454, p. 454: 'Jung, by his "modifications" has furnished psychoanalysis with a counterpart to the famous knife of Lichtenberg. He has changed the hilt, has inserted into it a new blade, and because the same trademark is engraved on it he requires of us that we regard the instrument as the former one.'
4 R. Barthes, 2007, *Il discorso amoroso. Seminario a l'École Pratique des Hautes Études 1974–1776, seguito da Frammenti di un discorso amoroso (inediti)*. Milano-Udine, Italy: Mimesis, p. 128.
5 *Ibid*., p. 489.
6 T. H. Ogden, 2008, *Rediscovering Psychoanalysis: Thinking and Dreaming, Learning and Forgetting*. London: Routledge.
7 See also S. Nacht, 1962, 'The curative factors in psycho-analysis', *International Journal of Psychoanalysis*, 43: 206–211, p. 210: 'No one can cure another if he has not a genuine desire to help him; and no one can have the desire to help unless he *loves*, in the deepest sense of the word'.
8 V. Chetrit-Vatine, 2014 [2012], *The Ethical Seduction of the Analytic Situation: The Feminine-Maternal Origins of Responsibility for the Other*. London: Routledge.
9 J. Kristeva, 1987, *In the Beginning Was Love: Psychoanalysis and Faith*. New York: Columbia University Press, p. 7.

M

MAESTRO. A hotel in Rome. After checking in, A., my travel companion, asks if they can serve him breakfast up in his room the next morning.

No, sir, unfortunately this service is not available.
How so? *Not* available?!
No, unfortunately …
Is there no way … ?
No, sir, I'm sorry …
(*Upon reflection*) Do you know what? A couple of days ago I happened to be talking to my wife about this … this thing about hotels not serving breakfast in your room. And you know what? She didn't want to believe me! SHE DID NOT WANT TO BELIEVE IT! And I kept telling her: 'That's the way it is!' And she goes: 'But that's not possible, nowadays … I DON'T BELIEVE IT … And where is this place? … And are you still going there?'

Witnessing this exchange, I was astonished. The disappointment had been conveyed through a civilized and humorous protest. A.'s wife, without knowing it, had been requested to act as a character who had only to say a few words, but was crucial in expressing his complaint in a form that would be effective and acceptable to everyone. Instead of irritating the clerk, A. made it seem like the only hotel where there is no breakfast room service is on Neptune.

In analysis, the play of characters can be equally useful to delicately address patients.

MANDALA. The record of a session, starting from anamnesis, if read as the analyst's interrupted or never-dreamed dream about the analysis it refers to, is a kind of mandala, or a microcosm that contains a perfect representation of the world. No longer an accessory, a secondary or a simple appendix to a *different* and more real scene, but a new, equally true, staging of the *same* scene.

MASK. During a session, a little girl plays with a mask by putting it on and taking it off. But the mask does not stay on as it does not have an elastic band. So the child asks the therapist if he has a rubber band. What she is really asking is, thanks to analysis, to give her the ability to adjust the distance from the object and so to be able to put on her mask by *herself*.

MASOCHISM. The pleasure the subject derives from the replica of the masochistic drama, when it is 'aesthetically' successful, could be the sublimative one of representation, a pleasure that in fact confirms the love of the object. The sense of masochism would be to revive the body by means of a compulsion to repeat understood not as a subservience to the death drive but as the work of 'somatic'/semiotic categorization and then of figurability. In retrospect, the oedipal fantasy would intervene in translating the masochistic fantasies in the body and/or would add up to them. From this angle, the repetition of trauma is never 'pure' repetition, and every episode tends to virtually metaphorize all the others in an attempt to make a concept out of them. Each new perverse scene would therefore represent a 'carrying out [...] in play'[1] of the perverse fantasy and would tend towards the 'highly enjoyable' experience of tragedy (expressions in inverted commas are quotes from Freud[2]). In my opinion, this could be the key to masochism.

MEDAL. S. arrives and fills me with hyperbolic praise because in the previous session she felt I helped her greatly. I am delighted, and I immediately think of Muttley, the cartoon character produced by Hanna-Barbera in 1968. Muttley is Dick Dastardly's dog. The two live in the period of World War I, and fight like heroes to intercept Yankee Doodle, a carrier pigeon that delivers messages to the enemy. Muttley does everything to earn Dick's approval, who with great satisfaction occasionally pins medals on the dog's chest (and if necessary he takes them away when Muttley, who is cowardly and is not very loyal, makes some major mistake). One could describe theirs as a love–hate relationship. Unlike in the original version, in the Italian dubbing Muttley speaks and his expression 'Medal, medal!' has become famous.[3]

Identifying myself with this likeable character, I willingly accept gratification. Cautiously, however, I also keep my distance – the medals can be revoked and in any case, they are made of cardboard. The affective climate then becomes even more intimate for the memory of something we loved and, more so because it was in the years of our childhood. Finally, I silently thank L. for making me feel good.

METALEPSIS. In narratology it indicates the transgression of the universes where the story is told.[4] For example, the narrator addresses the reader or, as in Julio Cortazar's *Continuity of the Parks*, at the end a character comes out of the pages of the book and stabs (!) the reader. The point of this metanarrative strategy is to denounce the naïve realism with which we look at things. The most natural of these short-circuits between worlds is the one between being awake and dreaming. By definition, the metaleptic device of psychoanalysis is the interpretation of transference. The subject is systematically displaced from the setting where he believed he was and finds out he has an 'amphibious' nature.

METAPSYCHOLOGY. If we mean Freudian metapsychology, it is sometimes confused by the French with the defence of their language and culture. In that case, for them it is a *shibboleth* of true psychoanalysis, and for others grist to the mill of chauvinism.

METONYMY. Julia Kristeva describes the process of birth of the psyche in the infant as the gradual settling of a feeling of deep revulsion for the mother's body. The maternal body becomes appalling to them, as will happen later, when they're adults, in the case of their own hair or nails as soon as they are detached from the body to which they belonged only a moment ago.

But one could say that the same disgust is caused by certain *mental* elements that we recognize as our own, but which we feel are separate. I am referring to all the various types of obsessive thoughts. The subject recognizes the obsessive idea as his own but wishes to eliminate it because he feels it as abject. He treats it like dirt he cannot erase and because of this he feels besieged, or feels its immanence as threatening and suffocating.

Based on the series of equivalences which I postulated between a mother's abject body, and the abjectness of one's own body and of one's own psychic elements, it is easy to see in obsession the collapse of the spacing or symbolizing function of metonymy. Like the languid fibres of a hyposthenic muscle, it no longer has the strength needed to move away from a disturbing stimulus. The *contact* that normally controls the momentum of the metonymic shift loses its leap and produces only a sterile series of attempts. Instead of releasing the subject from the object's slavery (like metaphor, metonymy is the agent of the slide from signifier to signifier which produces meaning) it generates a *metonymic delusion*.

MEXICO. After a trip to Mexico: 'Maybe it's the sun … the heat … something has changed … I feel as if … as if I haven't been coming for a long time'. I think to myself that, even though she's been turning up to sessions regularly, maybe it really feels like she *hasn't* been coming for a long time.

MIRROR-BODY. Sometimes seeing yourself looking at the analyst and seeing the analyst look at you at the beginning and end of the session is equivalent to being reflected in a *total* object. For some this is disturbing because it is as if it had the effect of prematurely forcing the reintrojection of one's own split mental aspects. It occurs when the patient is not yet ready to solve the relative disconnection between mind and body which is in some way at the bottom of all forms of mental suffering. Usually the problematic impulses are related to sexuality and seduction, that is to the libidinal and aggressive drives that are rooted in the body. The 'whole' vision of one's own as well as someone else's body awakens them much more than that of 'dematerialized' bodies reduced by the setting only to voices.

MOTHER TONGUE. Barthes: 'The writer is someone who plays with his mother's body'.[5]

MOURNING. The film *Extremely Loud and Incredibly Close*,[6] based on Jonathan Safran Foer's[7] novel of the same title, is moving. An 11-year-old boy with Asperger's syndrome grapples with unimaginable grief after the death of his father, whom he lost in the attack on the twin towers in New York. The film effectively shows the mental work involved in mourning, that is, the gradual acceptance of loss, making sense of the senseless trauma. We understand that the decisive element which made the process a success was the discreet yet attentive and empathetic presence of the mother.

MUSIC. Barthes:[8]

> When Charlotte plays the harpsichord, Werther forgets every dark idea; it calms him down, makes him breathe more freely, prevents him from 'planting a bullet in his head'. In the Charlotte that plays, the one that calms is the Mother; she takes the lover in her arms to cradle him; Werther resembles a sleepless baby who needs the body of his beloved to fall asleep: always accomodating, filtered, phrased, feeble, the (romantic) melody is really the substitute for his mother; whatever the expressive turns, no matter what it tells, its being is that of the Lullaby. The distressed subject is transported in it, suspended by a rhythmic body, which is neither inert nor busy: at the ready, weightless […] Music is always silent. It doesn't clutter me with any last word; it doesn't want to replace anything in my malaise (which is the best reason for exploring it further), it suspends it. It is an *epochè*, like the zero degree of all systems of meaning, which, instead, indiscreetly act to suppress in me the only freedom that matters to me today: to be delusional (*mainomai*: I'm lost, I'm in love) […] Soothed, busy with a refrain, the lover is similar to an autistic baby, able to repeat the music tunes and spend hours listening to the same aria: maybe because both of them make sure nothing changes.

This exemplary passage, which can only be quoted almost in its entirety, makes one reflect on how psychoanalysis has at times becoming hyper-rationalistic, and has neglected the sense of harmony and of the aesthetics of the encounter.

MYSTICISM. The thought of the great mystics can be useful, not to establish a mystical psychoanalysis – we would not know what to do with it – but to forge new concepts, to inspire new metaphors and to react thoroughly with a counter-loss to the sense of 'getting-lost' (*Verirrung*)[9] which, according to Heidegger, abstract thought produces with respect to reality.

There is, however, a kind of generative grammar of the psyche which renders all man-made forms of expression nothing but local dialects of a single national language. This is where the possibility of fertile transpositions is born.

Notes

1 S. Freud, 1924, 'The economic problem of masochism', *The Standard Edition of the Complete Psychological Works of Sigmund Freud*, vol. 19. London: The Hogarth Press, p. 162.
2 S. Freud, 1920, 'Beyond the pleasure principle', *The Standard Edition of the Complete Psychological Works of Sigmund Freud, vol. 19. London: The Hogarth Press*, pp. 1–64, p. 17.
3 www.youtube.com/watch?v=pHRg34eEAX0 (Accessed: August 20, 2018).
4 G. Civitarese, 2007, 'Metalessi ovvero retorica dell'interpretazione di transfert', *Rivista di Psicoanalisi*, 53:5–28.
5 R. Barthes, 1975, *The Pleasure of Text*. New York: Hill & Wang, p. 37.
6 S. Daldry (director), *Extremely Loud and Incredibly Close*, USA, 2011.
7 J. S. Foer, 2005, *Extremely Loud and Incredibly Close*. Boston, MA; New York: Houghton Mifflin Harcourt.
8 R. Barthes, 2007, *Il discorso amoroso. Seminario a l'École Pratique des Hautes Études 1974–1776, seguito da Frammenti di un discorso amoroso (inediti)*. Milano-Udine, Italy: Mimesis, pp. 592–593.
9 M. Heidegger, 2014 [2009], *Pensieri–guida. Sulla nascita della metafisica, della scienza contemporanea e della tecnica moderna*. Milano: Bompiani, p. 109.

N

NAILS. As a child, she would nibble at the hands and noses of her dolls, as if, she says, 'biting my own nails was no longer enough to keep me calm'.

NARRATION. The general function of the unconscious as a spontaneous activity of the mind is carried out in the creation of narratives. It could not be otherwise. That is why narratology is not only the scientific study of how stories are told but how in general we make sense of experience. In narratology a function is a 'transformation operator'. Beyond the objects and events, which can be variable, what counts in analysis is to identify the specific function that is activated because it corresponds to basic human emotions. Behind every function the analyst tries to decipher what is the unconscious (proto-)emotion that corresponds to it. Any narrative in a given relational context is read as the unconscious way of making sense of the experience lived in the present. Listening analytically means to have techniques for mapping the field of the relationship and intuiting where the patient is, in order to be able to meet her. But this is just a metaphor. Beyond the metaphor it means recognizing the unconscious expression of positive and negative emotions, getting an idea of how she responds, what helps her or what makes her hurt, trying to put yourself on the same wavelength. If, for example, a patient reacts to an interpretation by mentioning Hurricane Katrina, I deduce that I might have frightened her: 'meeting' her would then have the sense of modulating the level and intensity of my way of relating to her.

NEGATIVE CAPACITY. Heidegger's[1] volume *Discourse on Thinking* [*Gelassenheit*] can be read in the light of Bion's[2] essay 'Notes on memory and desire'. In addition to having a constant dialogue with

Kant, the two authors share an inspiration from Christian mysticism (Eckhartian, in particular: the expression *unio mystica* with respect to the concept of *unison/at-one-ment* is brought to mind), but in a detheologized and demythicized function.

The language of mysticism is transposed into the philosophical or psychoanalytic one. For the traditional categories, the effect is disruptive: a new lexicon and a new dictionary of concepts are introduced. Through a strenuous struggle with the word to express what is in fact ineffable, both authors make use of the mystic to nourish psychoanalytic thinking in the one case (the divine is replaced by the unconscious) and speculative in the other (instead of God, *lógos*). Finally, Bion and Heidegger arrive at the highest level of appreciation of thinking-dreaming in the case of the former and (through Hölderlin) of thinking-as-writing-poetry in the latter's case (the *Denken* to *Dichten* combination). Translated as 'abandonment' or 'releasement', *Gelassenheit* also means 'calm', 'tranquillity'. The term indicates a kind of 'quiet detachment' whose function is, again, to increase receptivity to the 'truth' of the unconscious or of Being. The ideal state of docile abandonment or submissive trust ('Faith', for Bion) is achieved through active renunciation of passions and desires.

The assumption is to 'let oneself go', a sort of of 'indifference to real life' – a concept that evokes the Bionian military precepts about the need to put the past behind us and to concentrate instead on what is happening in the present is echoed in Heidegger's criticism of the calculating thought and in his characterization of the meditative thought as a gathering 'on what lies close and what [...] is closest' and occurs in the 'here and now, here, on this patch of home ground; now, in the present hour of history'[3] –. In this way, Fabris writes,[4] keeping himself available and entrusted to it, man 'can relate to the burden of thought, to what cannot be thought of because it is before every thought'.

Discourse on Thinking – the German edition from 1959 – consists of two short texts. The first, corresponding to the title of the book, is an address given by the author in 1955, the second, 'Conversation on a country path about thinking', is drawn from conversations from 1944/45. Heidegger structures this second chapter in a way that anticipates Bion's trilogy *A Memoir of the Future*, like a three-voice dialogue between a scientist (S), a teacher (T) and a scholar (Sch). Below I quote an important fragment:

> S: In many respects it is clear to me what the word releasement should not signify for us. But at the same time, I know less and less what we are talking about. We are trying to determine the nature of thinking. What has releasement to do with thinking?
>
> T: Nothing if we conceive thinking in the traditional way as re-presenting. Yet perhaps the nature of thinking we are seeking is fixed in releasement (*ist in die Gelassenheit eingelassen*).
>
> S: With the best of will, I cannot re-present to myself this nature of thinking.
>
> T: Precisely because this will of yours and your mode of thinking as re-presenting prevent it.
>
> S: But then, what in the world am I to do?
>
> SCH: I am asking myself that too.
>
> T: We are to do nothing but wait (*warten*).[5]
> […]
>
> SCH: I'm not sure I understand what you say now.
>
> T: I don't understand it either, if by "understanding" you mean the capacity to represent what is put before us as if sheltered amid the familiar and so secured; for I, too, lack the familiar in which to place what I tried to say about openness as a region.[6]

The point is to get rid of one's mask as a subject, to get unused to will, to persevere in a sort of passivity, not to wait but to wait 'for something without knowing for what'.[7]

THE NEIGHBOUR I.

> I am going to kill my neighbour! … She said something horrible to me! … And I don't even have a way to avoid *her*, because of the way the house is … And *she* doesn't even realize just how much I cannot stand *her*![8]

THE NEIGHBOUR II. A. tells me for the umpteenth time about her neighbour who is hateful and bigoted. Then she asks me to explain some things to her. I remain silent. She becomes nervous and warns me: 'JUST WATCH ME "NEIGHBOURISING!"' The quick joke clarifies various perspectives of meaning. First of all, it reveals the reversibility of positions between herself and the neighbour as the ultimate incarnation of the world that she rejects, and therefore it is an ongoing process of re-introjection of split and projected psychic contents. One senses that, by transference, anyone who is near her can, in fact, be seen as 'the neighbour', and that her 'neighbour'-part is usually silent (as I was with her). Finally, 'playing the neighbour' is a way of getting close. In this way she gives voice to a livelier part of oneself, a part usually inhibited, shortens the distance and experiences a new intimacy.

NIGHT AND DAY. In January 2015, the New Museum in New York hosted a Chris Ofili[9] exhibition titled *Night and Day.* At one point you entered into a large room bathed in shadows. The visitor could just barely make out some large panels hanging on the walls. The sight adaptation to the darkness was not enough to distinguish the images that were painted. It was only by moving slowly that, with the slightest play of light, faint spotlights arranged artfully, the contours of large and disturbing figures could be captured, but never in their entirety. The system invented by Ofili thus revealed the unseen and aroused feelings of awe and reverence. This was not only due to the nature of the painted subjects, but because the extraordinary experience of interaction which the spectator underwent was itself a figure of a hopelessly lonely and precarious vision, like that of an inhabitant of the world of shadows.

In the same way, to grasp the visions of the unconscious, the encounter, always delicate and uncertain, must be realized, between a play of darkness and a cautious explorative movement, between renouncing the dazzling light of memories and opening up to the *experience* of remembering. To restoring faith in what disturbs us at first (the semi-darkness), what is almost irritating and would have us running the other way, promises to invoke impressive visions. From the absence of light comes the possibility of hallucinosis as of the most acute vision.

NIGHTMARE. If for Freud dreams have a natural tendency to transference, it is even more true for nightmares. When we wake up from a nightmare, we are hungry for meaning. The spontaneous impulse is to immediately wake someone up, if they are there, and tell them about it. The urgency is to find a container, a receptive mind capable of reverie. However, to drive away the fear and to go back to sleep, it is often enough to stretch out an arm and recover physical contact with another. It is clear then that dreaming, in the sense of giving meaning to things which in itself has a calming value, is first and foremost a dreaming *in* the body. We sense that physical contact (the touching of two bodies) is the prototype of any psychic containment and that it preserves for the whole life the same extraordinary power it had at birth. In accordance with our current way of theorizing its main therapeutic factors, analysis can be defined as a 'touching' cure just as much as a talking cure.

Notes

1 M. Heidegger, 1966 [1959], *Discourse on Thinking*. New York: Harper & Row.
2 W. R. Bion, 1967, 'Notes on memory and desire', *Psychoanalytic Forum*, 2:272–280.
3 Heidegger, *Discourse on Thinking*, cit., p. 47.
4 A. Fabris, 1998, 'Note', in: M. Heidegger, 1959, *L'abbandono*. Genova: il melangolo, p. 87.
5 Heidegger, *Discourse on Thinking*, cit., p. 62.
6 *Ibid.*, p. 65.
7 *Ibid.*, p. 68.
8 Play on words: in Italian, the third person singular (*lei*, she) is used as a formal way (and written with a capital 'L' as 'Lei') of saying 'you'. Therefore, here this could just as well mean: 'I don't even have a way to avoid *you*, because of the way the house is … And *you* don't' even realize just how much I cannot stand *you*'.
9 www.newmuseum.org/exhibitions/view/chris-ofili (Accessed: July 8, 2018).

O

O. As he admitted himself, Bions's O comes from Kant's thing-in-itself, which in turn was inspired by the *tò òn* from ancient Greek philosophy. A common mistake is to think of O as an entity located on this side the phenomenon, i.e. yes, unknowable but always situated within a human horizon. On the contrary, the Kantian distinction is between the narrowness of human knowledge and infinite knowledge or pure intellectual intuition which could belong to God. So, to say that O is unknowable is the same as saying that it can be known only in the human sense.

O (INFAMOUS). Sometimes I think that we should ask all analysts who study or are inspired by Bion, not to mention the concept of O for a few years. This bizarre idea of Bion, introduced to impose a phenomenological view of the facts of analysis and to stress the difference between emotional experience and intellectual knowledge, gives rise to the most absurd and hilarious interpretations.

OBSESSION. 'I'm not interested in writing short stories. Anything that doesn't take years of your life and drive you to suicide hardly seems worth doing': Cormac McCarthy in an article in *The Wall Street Journal*[1] a few years ago. This wonderful sentence is not only a precious poetic key to understanding the author's books, but could be used to distinguish between what is worth doing and what isn't in everyday life. If a film, a book of fiction or non-fiction does not have the intensity that only desperate obsession may have prompted in a talented writer or director, and if they do not reflect an obsession *of ours*, why bother with it? All great authors usually have this fire that devours them and pushes them to create.

The obsession must be so violent that it does not leave much space for anything else. In fact, we see that each of them does nothing but deal from start to finish on their own creative parabola with one and only one great idea and not much more. This superb monotony of themes and style reveals how high are the walls of the secret prison where thought is generated. And yet, even if it holds the subject captive, the obsession (the siege) serves as a container for anguish. The figure of suicide explicitly evoked by McCarthy refers here to the depressive void which nurtures creativity and from which obsessiveness sees a way out.

OBSESSIVE NEUROSIS. Obsessive neurosis could be renamed conceptual/ideational or 'abstract-ive' neurosis, in the sense that the subject seems to become nothing but thought. Their struggle against the risk of being overwhelmed by uncontrollable emotional states is demonstrated by the content of the obsessive impulse, which is often to harm another or to harm oneself. In the compulsion to think, we can see the superhuman effort aimed at interposing a distance of safety between oneself and these emotions. In essence, to detach oneself from one's own body. Which is – it goes without saying – impossible.

Notes

1 J. Jurgensen, 'Hollywood's Favorite Cowboy', *The Wall Street Journal*, November 20, 2009.

P

PADDLE BOAT I.

Shall we go for a swim together?
Let's go.
Do you want to take a paddle boat?
I won't be able to get on it.
Oh NOOO … come on!

He gets up and brings all his excess kilos to inspect the yellow paddle boat, then comes back and settles down lazily on the sunbed under a parasol.

OUT OF THE QUESTION! … the keel is raised.
Were you not able to get on?
No.
Is there no boarding ladder?
No.
Are you sure?
Yes … I saw it.
There is none.
There is none.
None?
Exactly.
Sure. Tomorrow we could go to another beach.
Let's go somewhere else.
Maybe I'll go there … *by myself.*
Well, yeah, sure … you could go there … by yourself.
We could go on *holidays* … alone.

Sitting on the sunbed, her head bowed, she studies the sand baked by the sun where her feet rest. He moves away to take two steps along the shoreline. When he turns around, he addresses her (kindly):

If you want, later I can bring you on the paddle boat around five o'clock … The sun won't be as strong then … I'll put on a shirt …

Meanwhile, a street vendor comes over.

Do you want a watch from Mustafa?!

This time she doesn't reply.

PADDLE BOAT II. Being a father is difficult. I read this scene in a story written by R* when he was just over fifteen years old.

> Leonardo woke up. His vision was blurry. His father was lying on the sunbed next to him. Giorgio was digging a hole under the parasol.
>
> What time is it?
>
> The sea looked like a puddle of boiling water. The breeze smoothed the waves. The white sky was sinking in the waters.
>
> Leo – murmured his father – I thought I saw one of your friends from last year.
>
> Where?
>
> They're over there.
>
> A group of teenagers were about to go on a paddle boat. Leo remined unmoved.
>
> We could go as well if you want suggested the father.
>
> How many times, as a child, had he begged his father to go on a paddle boat to enjoy the thrill of gripping the helm? Thousands. As a teenager? Half a dozen. And every time father and son reached the buoy, far from everything and everyone, Remo Toscani, the lawyer, pronounced the fateful word: university. His father was obsessed with it. He was obsessed with the faculty, with the location. He wanted his son to secure a future, to make the right choice.
>
> Leonardo felt observed. All his father ever did was walk around him, sniff around, and try to guess his thoughts.
>
> Leonardo felt like he was being hunted down.

The paddle boat trips with his father became more and more rare, only to finally become extinct. Now, after all that, he did not even need him to put his hand around the helm. He was sixteen. He was grown up. He could go on the pedal boat alone. In his oppressed state of mind, with a father who is a lawyer and a mother who is a judge, all he longed for was to hoist his sails and become a pirate.

To rebel.

The wind in his face. The prow breaking on the waves. Having the impression of navigating to infinity. Without a thought. Without a word.

PARADIGM. An old colleague gives out to me for wanting to talk about many (too many) concepts which sound new to him. I would pretend to make him accept that everything he believed he knew for a lifetime is outdated today. He reminds me of a Bion's idea that something which cannot be recognized and assimilated by the other is not true. However, endless and fruitless discussions arise from ignorance of the Kuhnian concept of paradigm and from the desecrating depiction that Feyerabend has given about the workshop of science.

When defining a new paradigm, a new vocabulary of words and concepts is used. Therefore, you should be aware of the problems affecting translation. Different paradigms are immeasurable among them, and only for the 'bilinguals' do they admit a certain translatability. But even they must give up on the hope for a perfect translation. On the one hand, this requires a work of mourning. On the other hand, in the successful cases, you gain a new understanding of the object.

PARANORMAL ACTIVITY. 'We used to go to the cinema together. One of my favourite films was *Paranormal Activity.*[1] A little girl could spit fire from her eyes and set things on fire … What do you think about my relationship with my parents?' I said:

> You told me before that today you wished … to focus (*mettere a fuoco*, in Italian; literally: to set on fire) on some details of your relationship with your father … maybe the answer is already there …. By replacing the girl in the film who spurted fire with her eyes in anger …

In analysis, what sounds real is usually unexpected and surprising. However, sometimes the truth seems banal.

PARENTHESIS. In the text of the session, S. put all the sentences he had addressed to the patient in parenthesis, as it is common to do for any marginal notes. In the text of the patient's discourse, instead, he put in brackets dozens of lines of theoretical explanation. A double demonstration of withdrawal from the relationship, in the first case by deficiency and in the second by excess.

PARTHENOGENESIS. To evoke the extraordinary creative power of the dream at the end of the volume on Swann's loves, Proust uses the image of parthenogenesis: the most fertile among all the ways of generating a new living form.

PERFECTNESS. For Emily Dickinson the aurora is the heavenly vault's effort to simulate a perfectness unbeknown to itself.[2] According to this inspired image, perfection in analysis would be the maximum amount of spontaneity made possible by the work of the Unconscious, to the point of unconsciousness.

PERFORMATIVITY. In reading Bion it is typical to suddenly pass from the level of the most abstruse theory and illogical use of mathematical symbols to clinical vignettes (as in certain American cities, when you walk across a street and everything is changed all of a sudden). Hatred, jealousy, paranoia, violent emotions (it is the *power* of an emotion rather than its character that determines its destiny, he writes), feelings of frustration, phantasies, come back onto the stage, as if they had been excluded for too long. In a completely involuntary way the transition produces the surprising coincidence of statement and enunciation we refer to as the concept of performativity. Suddenly we understand and sigh with relief. We verify the accuracy of Bion's essential theoretical insight consisting in putting emotion at the core of psychoanalysis as the element that gives meaning to existence. We empathize with patients forced to live in worlds that are dramatically devoid of it, we savour the sense of vitality that finally seems to have found us again.

PERSONA. This is a reference to Ingmar Bergman's film of the same title. The scene where a boy wakes up and tries to touch the face of his mother as big as the wall of a room is worth more than words to understand the meaning of concepts such as dream screen and aesthetic conflict.

PERSONS AND THINGS. Roberto Esposito's[3] essay *Le persone e le cose* [*Persons and Things*] should be read by all analysts. From a non-psychological perspective, he reminds us that, for example as regards to Roman law, no one ever becomes a person once and for all, and that one's status as a person is always the fruit of a continuous negotiation. You can gain it but you can also lose it. It is no coincidence that a mask (in Latin, 'persona') adheres to the face while still remaining separate from it.

Against every naïve, essentialistic conception of the subject, Esposito awakens us to the notion of sociality, identified with language, as the ground from which we could never tear ourselves away because we would die. In this regard, for example, the classic studies of Marcel Mauss on psychogenic death come to mind, as well as those of Peter Fonagy on the violence arising from shame as an extreme and destructive attempt to resuscitate the gaze of the other.

While listening to S. telling me about her obligation to her father to pay back the money he had given her to buy a car, I remembered Esposito's essay and the way he describes the credit–debtor relationship as one of those that can degrade you from the status of a person and reduce you to that of a thing. It is clear that the association could convey the idea that the relationship between the two was not particularly peaceful. That is clear, but it also reminded me of the role of money between me and her as an element of the analytic setting and once again problematized the ambiguity necessary in the analytic relationship, which is always in tension between truth and fiction.

PLAY. Ttransformation in play, a formula proposed by Antonino Ferro, is more readily understandable than that of transformation in dream. Everybody understands that we accept the suspension of disbelief in a game, the fact of being completely immersed in it and contributing to pushing it forward in a certain way, while not everybody reads dreams in the same way, for example as a shared dream in the here and now.

POETRY. Ezra Pound writes: 'Music begins to athrophy when it departs *too* far from the dance. Poetry begins to athrophy when it gets too far from music.'[4] For the transitive property, writing poetry is dancing. The value of poetry is in action, in the body.

PRESSURE. In physics, pressure and temperature are the two factors that lead to the critical point of the phase transition. In analysis they could be, respectively, the emotional warmth or involvement the analyst shows on the one hand, and the tension that he imposes on the patient every time he offers a different perspective on things on the other.

PROBLEMS. Sometimes it might help us to understand what we do if for a second we simply stop using terms like truth, insight, transformation, mind growth, subjectivation, and the like, and instead use the word *problem*. At each session in one way or another the patient brings us a problem, which is of an emotional nature – this is our area of intervention, not, for example, that of concrete reality. They express it either in a clear and direct or an allusive or allegorical form, in words or in silence. The point becomes to define the problem and find a solution using the same rhetorical resources and the same narrative genres proposed by the patient.

PSYCHOANALYSIS I. The analyst and the patient like the two teenagers in the old Tim (a telecommunications company) ad promoting the *Duetto* offer, who keep asking 'Do you love me? But how much … ?!'[5]

PSYCHOANALYSIS II. The analyst and the patient like Bruce Willis in *The Sixth Sense*[6] as a (unlikely) psychologist and the boy who refused to speak. If he says something that touches him, he suggests to the kid that he take a few steps forward towards him; if not, that he move back.

PSYCHOANALYSIS III. The analyst and the patient like two Geomag[7] pieces continuously striving to turn to find the best position to attract each other but often only succeeding in repelling one other.

PSYCHOANALYSIS IV. Can we still define psychoanalysis as a theory that limits itself to chanting Freud from the first half of the last century, as if nothing has happened since then? Is it still possible to use the concept of drives as if they were not, as he defined them, a kind of mythology? Is there a point in reducing masochism and human destructiveness to the death drive? Or paranoia to hidden homosexuality? If Freud was reborn today, would he go to his most zealous followers or would he be attracted to those in whom he would recognize his own spirit of research and courage similar to his own?

PSYCHOANALYSIS V. An exercise in systematic self-criticism of enunciation? It is born from the fact that, as Barthes[8] notes, though we know it from Bion onwards, if we take seriously the concepts of the unconscious as a psychoanalytic function of personality and of the waking-dream thought, 'the unconscious is everywhere, and not "at the bottom"; it is there from the moment an act of enunciation is made'.

PSYCHOPATHY. Patients with antisocial tendencies typically arouse in the therapist both fascination and fear. This mixture of feelings, too different to be unified into a coherent (affective) concept of the other is the clearest mirror of the anti-sociability from which the object suffered. That is to say that, at the time, the object was not able to identify enough with the subject, but, instead, seduced and rejected him inconsistently. In treatment, the analyst's inner life as a place of the analytic field becomes the ground, hopefully more favourable, where once again the battle of the aesthetic conflict is fought, and all efforts are made to try and win it.

PSYCHOSIS. From the record of a session: 'A. arrives 5 minutes late. I open the door and see that right after her B., my old psychotic patient, sneaked into the office. I excuse myself to A. and make sure to get B. out the door. A. asks me, "Did she get the wrong time? I found her sitting outside. She seemed to know me and when I came in she came in right behind me"'. If we read all of this as the narration of a dream, we could not help thinking that something belonging to A.'s psychotic personality has been actively expelled from the analytic field and is trying to get in. Maybe the same one who, by mistake, arrived five minutes late.

Notes

1 C. Minihan (director), *Paranormal Activity*, Canada, 2011.
2 E. Dickinson, 1960, *The Complete Poems of Emily Dickinson*. New York: Little, Brown & Company, p. 465.
3 R. Esposito, 2015, *Le persone e le cose*. Torino: Einaudi.
4 E. Pound, 1991, *ABC of Reading*. London: Faber & Faber, p. 14.
5 www.youtube.com/watch?v=T5fbQZjdE6g (Accessed: July 8, 2018).
6 M. Night Shyamalan (director), *The Sixth Sense*, USA, 1999.
7 For the word 'aimant', which in French means both 'lover' (as an adjective) and 'magnet' (as a noun), see R. Barthes, 2007, *Il discorso amoroso. Seminario a l'École Pratique des Hautes Études 1974–1776, seguito da Frammenti di un discorso amoroso (inediti)*. Milano-Udine, Italy: Mimesis, p. 262.
8 *Ibid*., p. 500.

Q

QUESTIONS. While holding seminars and conferences around the world, I realized that often the questions that irritatate are the most useful ones because they are either naïve or provocative. Such questions puzzle and push you to think, or rather to slowly digest the little emotional catastrophe that they sometimes produced. One should always be grateful to those who have the courage to ask them.

R

RAGE. To get an idea of it, the amazing fight scene between Stark and Hulk in the movie *Avengers: Age of Ultron*.[1]

RESONANCE. *Knight of Cups* by Terence Malick,[2] a director I admire a lot, as usual shows charming images, but surprisingly I find it cold and it does not stir up the slightest emotion in me. My engagement is exclusively intellectual. It thus seems a meaningless exercise. It does, however, help to understand the value of *emotions* as a sign of a resonance effect (unison, sharing) in action. Resonance is a 'way of painful or jubilatory amplification', writes Barthes,[3] (while complaining that it has not been considered by any discourse, and 'especially the psychoanalytical one'. Had he read Bion, perhaps he would have held a different opinion).

Feeling a bit of resentment towards one of my cinema idols because of the disappointment suffered after seeing his latest work, I think about how the word *resentment*, which is so similar to the word resonance, but as far as a synonym of rancour, has such a negative connotation. But one need only think for a moment to understand why: unlike the former, the latter word does not refer to an isolated self but to a self in relation to the other.

However, the story does not end there. A friend whom I told about my sense of disillusionment, said to me: 'And if the purpose of the director was precisely to make the spectator experience the same sense of futility as the protagonist?' Having found his interpretation to have 'resonance' with me, I felt my resentment subside somewhat. Or let's say that I put it aside.

REVERIE. There is a lot of talk about reveries, and the more you talk about it, the less you understand what it is. I find that an essential point is easily lost, namely, that the reverie assumes value within the intersubjective conception that Bion has of psychoanalysis, by reference to the central concept of the waking-dream thought, to the criticism of the primary process/secondary process binary opposition, and to the unconscious as a psychoanalytic function of personality. It is therefore a mistake to reduce reverie to a countertransference phenomenon. At best, we would compare it to a countertransference dream: simply a dream with your eyes open. In line with this, we would read it with the claim to decipher it to get to the hidden 'true' thoughts. As you can see, it has nothing to do with the idea of a intersubjective analytic third or that of the analytic field.

REVERSAL OF PERSPECTIVE. As I distractedly observe the landscape, at some point I think the taxi driver who is taking me to the hotel has to be completely crazy because he keeps on overtaking everyone on the right (!) Then I shake myself awake from my open-eyed dream and realize that we just left Gatwick behind.

REVERSIBILITY. Merleau-Ponty describes a sensory reversibility with respect to the intersubjective constitution of the individual. In the metaphor of the analytic field, he gives an account of the mutual interdependence of all the elements that are co-present at a given moment. However, it is still difficult to get out from the spontaneous vision of two entities separated by a void, like monads. It is still too abstract. It would be different if we used the metaphor of the human body, of which we have a concrete experience, and how various organs touch and influence each other in a variety of ways: physical, hormonal, neuroelectric, etc. If we then translate the physical elements into psychic elements, we return to the Kleinian and Meltzerian idea of internal objects engaged in ceaseless interaction. On a clinical level, reversibility means that an emotion is never one-way; it never belongs only to one or the other of the components of the couple.

RHYTHM. I have always found this sentence of Winnicott's[4] illuminating where he talks about the meaning of music-as-container of the most primitive anxieties:

> Belonging to this feeling of helplessness [at birth] is the intolerable nature of experiencing something without any knowledge

> whatever of when it will end. […] It is for this reason fundamentally that form in music is so important. *Through form, the end is in sight from the beginning.*

These lines came to my mind when I subsequently came across a chapter in another book by Agamben, *The Man Without Content*, which deals with rhythm and is entitled 'The original structure of the work of art'. The *incipit* is flashy. Agamben quotes Hölderlin: 'Everything is rhythm, the entire destiny of man is one heavenly rhythm, just as every work of art is one rhythm, and everything swings from the poetizing lips of the god'.[5] Then the author wonders wherein consists this original character of the work of art which the poet assigns to rhythm. So, making reference to ancient philosophy he assimilates rhythm to the concept of '*structure*, schema, as opposed to elementary and inarticulate matter'.[6] The original being of any work of art would simply be ῥυθμός ('structure').[7] But what structure is in question here? Not structure as number but as 'ουσία, the principle of presence that opens and maintains the work of art in its original space'.[8] The term 'rhythm' comes from the Greek ῥέω, to pass, to flow. Whatever flows, flows in time. But into this unstoppable flow of linear time, impersonal and unclaimed, rhythm bursts like:

> a split and a stop. Thus in a musical piece, although it is somehow in time, we perceive rhythm as something that escapes the incessant flight of instants and appears almost as the presence of an atemporal dimension in time. In the same way, when we are before a work of art or a landscape bathed in the light of its own presence, we perceive a stop in time, as though we were suddenly thrown into a more original time. […] but this being arrested is also a being-outside, an *ek-stasis* in a more original dimension […] it is the original ecstasy that opens for man the space of his world.[9]

If I understand Agamben correctly, I would say that this is a question of identity and difference. Rhythm takes us out of ourselves, immersed as we are in the unnoticed flow of time, and by making us rediscover this crucial dimension it constitutes us as subjects. Rhythm roots us in the consciousness of time as the original domain of our being. In this, the echoes of Heidegger are obvious.

In order to explore further Agamben's suggestions, it is useful to read them in the light of the beautiful book, *Listening*, by Jean-Luc Nancy.[10] In this study he perhaps clarifies better the sense of rhythm as a 'continual differing from oneself'. Nancy writes,

> Perhaps we should thus understand the child who is born with his first cry as himself being – his being or his subjectivity – the sudden expansion of an echo chamber, a vault where what tears him away and what summons him resound at once, setting in vibration a column of air, of flesh, which sounds at its apertures: body and soul of some one new and unique.

For the human being, any seeing is seeing oneself seeing[11] and any hearing is hearing oneself hear. And thus openness to the world is established and the space for interiority is created. But if there is a 'rhythm' of seeing, this notion becomes even more pregnant when we consider listening. Seeing is already compromised by association with the rational pole of being (θεωρέιν means 'to look', 'to see'), with representation – and it is on the centrality of representation that Freud erected his theoretical edifice. Hearing, however, is still further beyond language. It has more to do with sense than with meaning. More to do with the body than with the intellect. Rhythm cuts out strips of time and in doing so subjectivizes it. Furthermore, it introduces a sense of space. Only time makes it possible for the spaces which typesetters place between words to become effective in constructing the meaning of the sentence. Technically this is called 'spacing'. The word is an addition to time and space, or rather, to duration which makes itself into space. Rhythm, writes Nancy, 'separates the succession of the linearity of the sequence or length of time: it bends time to give it to time itself, and it is in this way that it folds and unfolds a "self"'.[12] And he wonders, 'isn't the subject itself the starting of time in both values of the genitive: it opens it and it is opened by it? Isn't the subject the attack of time?'[13]

The notion of rhythm returns insistently when we find ourselves faced with the key theoretical crux of contemporary psychoanalysis, the unrepresentable: that is, the dimension of sense that both precedes and then accompanies linguistic signification, but which is not susceptible of any kind of translation that is not essentially intermodal (from one medium to another). It so happens that I have addressed this on at least three occasions: in relation to aesthetic conflict, in a chapter of *The Violence of Emotions*,[14] in the essay on Ferro entitled, appositely, 'Spacings',[15] and lastly in a recent study on masochism.[16] In the last of these, the concept of rhythm becomes the keystone of an attempt at an alternative theorization of masochism from the starting point of Freud's annotations in two of his three key essays on this subject, in 'Beyond the pleasure principle' and 'The economic problem of masochism'. In these wonderful works Freud gets to grips with the enigma of pleasure in pain:

> It seems that in the series of feelings of tension we have a direct sense of the increase and decrease of amounts of stimulus, and it cannot be doubted that there are pleasurable tensions and unpleasurable relaxations of tension. The state of sexual excitation is the most striking example of a pleasurable increase of stimulus of this sort, but it is certainly not the only one.
>
> Pleasure and unpleasure, therefore, cannot be referred to an increase or decrease of a quantity (which we describe as 'tension due to stimulus'), although they obviously have a great deal to do with that factor. It appears that they depend, not on this quantitative factor, but on some characteristic of it which we can only describe as a qualitative one. If we were able to say what this qualitative characteristic is, we should be much further advanced in psychology. Perhaps it is the rhythm, the temporal sequence of changes, rises and falls in the quantity of stimulus. We do not know.[17]

If it is a question of rhythm and not of absolute values, this also means that the first moment of 'unpleasure' at the increase of tension is nevertheless a component of the pleasure, and that every pleasure can be called a negative pleasure.

A further extraordinarily fertile suggestion about rhythm can be found in Nietzsche.[18] In an aphorism devoted to the origin of poetry he speaks about the power of rhythm 'that reorganizes all the atoms of a sentence', and constrains not only the body to a certain cadence of movements, but the soul itself, and even 'the souls of the gods', enabling us to draw closer to their ear and almost oblige them, so to speak, to keep time with us and receive our prayer. As Nietzsche observes, 'even the wisest of us occasionally becomes a fool for rhythm, if only insofar as he *feels* a thought to be *truer* when it has a metric form and presents itself with a divine hop, skip and jump'.[19]

RILKE. In a letter of dazzling beauty sent to Margot Sizzo, dated April 12, 1923, Rilke addresses the essence of the aesthetics of the sublime:

> More and more in my life and in my work, I am guided by the effort to correct our old repressions, which have removed and gradually estranged from us the mysteries out of whose abundance our lives might become truly infinite. It is true that these mysteries are dreadful, and people have always drawn away from them. But where can we find anything sweet and glorious that would never wear *this* mask, the mask of the dreadful? Life – and we know nothing else – isn't life itself dreadful? But as soon as we acknowledge its dreadfulness (not as opponents: what kind of match could we be for it?), but somehow with a confidence that this very dreadfulness may be something completely *ours*, though something that is just now too great, too vast, too incomprehensible for our learning hearts – : as soon as we accept life's most terrifying dreadfulness, at the risk of perishing from it (i.e. from our own Too-much!) – : then an intuition of blessedness will open up for us and, at this cost, will be ours. Whoever does not, sometime or other, give his full consent, his full and *joyous* consent, to the dreadfulness of life, can never take possession of the unutterable abundance and power of our existence; can only walk on its edge, and one day, when the judgement is given, will have been neither alive nor dead. To show the *identity* of dreadfulness and bliss, these two faces on the same divine head, indeed this one *single* face, which just presents itself this way or that,

according to our distance from it or the state of mind in which we perceive it – : this is the true significance and purpose of the Elegies and the Sonnets to Orpheus.[20]

ROLL. I'm on my way to the office. I go on foot to get some exercise and reduce the slight corpulence that has bothered me for some time. I'm a bit anxious because I realize that I might be late, maybe I would find the patient waiting for me, we would have to get the elevator together and the whole thing might be awkward for both of us. In a fraction of a second I SEE myself roll (!) downhill like a rubber Michelin man. The street slopes down slightly and in my waking dream I tell myself that I would get there faster! I can't help but laugh at the ingenious solution that transforms a little defect for which I get mocked at home, into an unexpected advantage. I reassure myself that humour is a sign of health at a time when I happen to be upset by some physical annoyances. Then, little by little, other interpretations come to mind. I think of possible meanings of rolling: rolling on the floor laughing, rolling around in bed (with A.?!?), rolling towards the last station …

RUBBER BAND. I was delighted to discover that in one of his lectures Alessandro Baricco comments upon the famous passage from Proust about the digger wasp. The passage is worth quoting in full:

> There is a species of hymenoptera observed by Fabre, the burrowing wasp, which in order to provide a supply of fresh meat for her offspring after her own decease, calls in the science of anatomy to amplify the resources of her instinctive cruelty, and, having made a collection of weevils and spiders, proceeds with marvellous knowledge and skill to pierce the nerve-centre on which their power of locomotion (but none of their other vital functions) depends, so that the paralysed insect, beside which she lays her eggs, will furnish the larvae, when hatched, with a docile, inoffensive quarry, incapable either of flight or of resistance, but perfectly fresh for the larder: in the same way Françoise had adopted, to minister to her unfaltering resolution to render the house uninhabitable to any other servant, a series of stratagems so cunning and so pitiless that, many years later, we discovered that if we had

> been fed on asparagus day after day throughout that summer, it was because their smell gave the poor kitchen-maid who had to prepare them such violent attacks of asthma that she was finally obliged to leave my aunt's service.[21]

The passage stretches like a rubber band and then bounces back and closes the circle. This is how any effective narrative works. It is the logic of pleasure, linked to the qualitative element of the *rhythm* with which the tension increases and then fizzles out. But a secret that not everyone knows is *how* to read Proust: *with strict compliance to punctuation*. Proust's sentence is like a metronome that forces the reader to re-align with time. Of course, you can also read it without respecting the pauses, but then it's like living a life with a false Self or a life of inauthenticity: the poetry is lost.

Notes

1 J. Whedon (director), *Avengers: Age of Ultron*, USA, 2015.
2 T. Malick (director), *Knight of Cups*, USA, 2015.
3 R. Barthes, 2007, *Il discorso amoroso. Seminario a l'École Pratique des Hautes Études 1974–1776, seguito da Frammenti di un discorso amoroso (inediti)*. Milano-Udine, Italy: Mimesis, p. 236.
4 D. W. Winnicott, 1984, *Through Pediatrics to Psychoanalysis*. London: Karnac Books, p. 184 (emphasis added).
5 G. Agamben, 1994, *The Man without Content*. Stanford, CA: Stanford University Press, 1999, p. 94.
6 *Ibid.*, p. 97.
7 *Ibid.*, p. 98.
8 *Ibid.*
9 *Ibid.*, pp. 99–100.
10 J.-L. Nancy, 2002, *Listening*. New York: Fordham University Press, 2007, pp. 17–18.
11 See V. Magrelli, 2002, *Vedersi vedersi. Modelli e circuiti visivi nell'opera di Paul Valéry*. Torino: Einaudi.
12 Nancy, *Listening*, cit., p. 17.
13 *Ibid.*, p. 75.
14 G. Civitarese, 2013 [2011], *The Violence of Emotions: Bion and Post-Bionian Psychoanalysis*. London: Routledge.
15 A. Ferro and G. Civitarese, 2015, *The Analytic Field and Its Transformations*. London: Karnac.
16 G. Civitarese, 2018, *Sublime Subjects: Aesthetic Experience and Intersubjectivity in Psychoanalysis*. London: Routledge.

17 S. Freud, 1924, 'The economic problem of masochism', *The Standard Edition of the Complete Psychological Works of Sigmund Freud*, vol. 19. London: The Hogarth Press, p. 160.
18 F. Nietzsche, 2001, *The Gay Science*. Cambridge: Cambridge University Press, p. 84.
19 *Ibid.*, pp. 85–86.
20 R. M. Rilke, 2009, *Duino Elegies and Sonnets to Orpheus*. New York: Mariner Book, pp. 222–223.
21 M. Proust, 1928, *Swann's Way.* Translated by C. K. Scott Moncrieff and T. Kilmartin, revised by D. J. Enright. New York: The Modern Library, p. 173.

S

SALVO.[1] A handsome,young actress from Pescara, Sara Serraiocco, plays Rita, the blind sister of a criminal who a killer from an opposing faction, Salvo (Saleh Bakri), comes to murder in his own house. He is going to kill Rita as well, but witnessing that she, trembling with fear, is suddenly able to see again, he feels a wave of pity for her. Rita is not the only one who miraculously regains sight as a result of a violent emotion; it happens to Salvo, too. Up to this point he has shown only the bestial and ruthless prowess of a dehumanized predator. One could say that the key moment of the film is in this sublime act of *agnition*.

SAMBA. The analyst should have the (wise) lightness recommended by Italo Calvino in his *If on a Winter's Night a Traveller*, the ability to subtract weight and stone-like quality from language and to bring an indirect way of looking at reality, but which would be at the same time accurate, rapid, visible, manifold, and coherent. By this I mean the ability to weave with the patient a 'happy' conversation and adapt to his awkwardness without even noticing it.

What brought on this train of thought was the memory of the high school birthday parties from the late '70s. Carlos Santana's 'Samba pa ti' was very much in at that time. A demonic song. It starts off slowly giving you the impression that you'll be able to handle it, but then it speeds up inexorably. A nightmare, if it weren't for A., my classmate: with a sinuous and sensual body, she graciously adapted to her partner's pace, even the clumsiest one. A clear example, I would say today, of how in a unison which is at the same time psychological and physical it is possible to strengthen in the other a sense of agency which is still rather fragile.

SCIENCE. No other 'science' lives in writing the way psychoanalysis does. It is a striking proof of its amphibious nature. Certainly not a science, perhaps somewhere *between* empirical science and literature, and yet closer to a hermeneutic phenomenology.

SEATTLE. A few days after I came back from the 10th international conference on 'Evolving British Object Relations' in Seattle, where I was the main speaker, I received a very nice letter and a drawing (Figure 6) from Caron Harrang, the colleague who organized the meeting:

> Dear Giuseppe,
>
> I also had an experience immediately following the conference that echoed the impact of the conference including, among other things, our conversation about transference/countertransference and field theory that I'll share with you to illustrate just how much the experience affected me.
>
> [...] I am more than satisfied with the conference. It was for me pure joy in how it came to fruition. Dana and I have heard from so many people how much they valued the experience starting out with The Art of Reverie (there were 30 people there from the general public) and continuing throughout the weekend. So, yes, a very rewarding experience for me.
>
> On Sunday immediately following the conference I decided to go kayaking from my brother's house on Lake Washington (in Kirkland) to get some exercise and relax after an intense couple of days. It was later in the afternoon, around 4:30 pm, when I paddled the mile and a quarter across the lake (see attached map). When I got to the Seattle side, feeling very happy to be out on the water and musing about the conference, I decided to go north along the shore before turning back and heading for home. In my mind, I intended to make a triangle route rather than a straight over and back paddle as I've done before.
>
> After paddling north for a third of a mile or so, I turned around and sighted on a patch of green grass across the lake, thinking that it was a park I was well familiar with a bit north of my brother's dock on the Kirkland side of the lake. By this time it was twilight and very beautiful, but not yet dark. I was still very much engaged with many thoughts about the weekend, particularly a sense that my psychoanalytic orientation is shifting and opening up as well as forging new friendships, such as ours.

So, I paddled back across the lake to the green patch of grass thinking it was a park I knew, only to find when I got there that it looked unfamiliar and I realized I wasn't where I thought I would be. Still, I reasoned that if I turned south and went along the shoreline I'd soon run into my brother's dock. By this time, however, it was fully dark and I could only see the houses close to the shore.

The further I went, the more unfamiliar the shoreline looked with no sight of my brother's dock and home on the hillside above. Hmm? At a certain point, after going quite a ways, I realized *I had no idea where I was or how to get back to familiar territory.* So, I pulled my kayak out of the water and approached a house near the shore where I saw some lights. I found a house where a family was gathered watching TV and went to their backdoor and called out, 'Hello'. From inside an older man looked in my direction and said, 'Who is it?' Eventually, the whole family and their dog came outside and I explained my situation. 'Where am I?' I inquired.

The family told me that I was in Juanita Bay, which is a fair distance from where I thought I was and needed to be to get back to my brother's home. They pointed out the lights of Kirkland in the distance, which I used to orient toward in heading back to the now very dark area where my brother's house and dock were located. As I paddled back toward familiar territory, I couldn't help wondering if my getting a bit lost and ending up in a new place mirrored my experience of the conference. A kind of somatic reverie or waking dream reflecting my sense of finding myself in a new place unexpectedly. And, even as I was now worried that my family would be wondering where I was and possibly worried, I couldn't help noticing how beautiful it was to be out on the lake at night with just a hint of moonlight.

In the meantime, my brother had put a lantern out on the end of his dock, hoping I'd see it and know that is where I needed to go to get home. When I saw it I recognized the dock and quickly made my way to shore. By this time, the Sheriff's Marine Department had been called and a rescue boat deployed to look for me, but that's another story. The search was quickly called off and the evening ended with a family dinner and much storytelling.

I'm glad you enjoyed the wine and hope that the experience of the conference was good for you too.

Warm wishes,
Caron Harrang, LICSW, FIPA

This delightful letter – it is not true that with e-mails one forgets how to write – depicts very well, as does the author in retrospect, the sense of alienation but also of adventure and discovery that you experience when you agree to go into territories hitherto unexplored.

SECONDARY SCHOOL. 'It seems a bit too much like high school in here!' L. reproached me pleasantly. I thought she meant that my way of addressing her was too intellectual. Months later, while listening to another patient whose session was just before hers, the episode came back to me. However this time I thought that my high school years had been rather happy. I then realized that my first interpretation of her

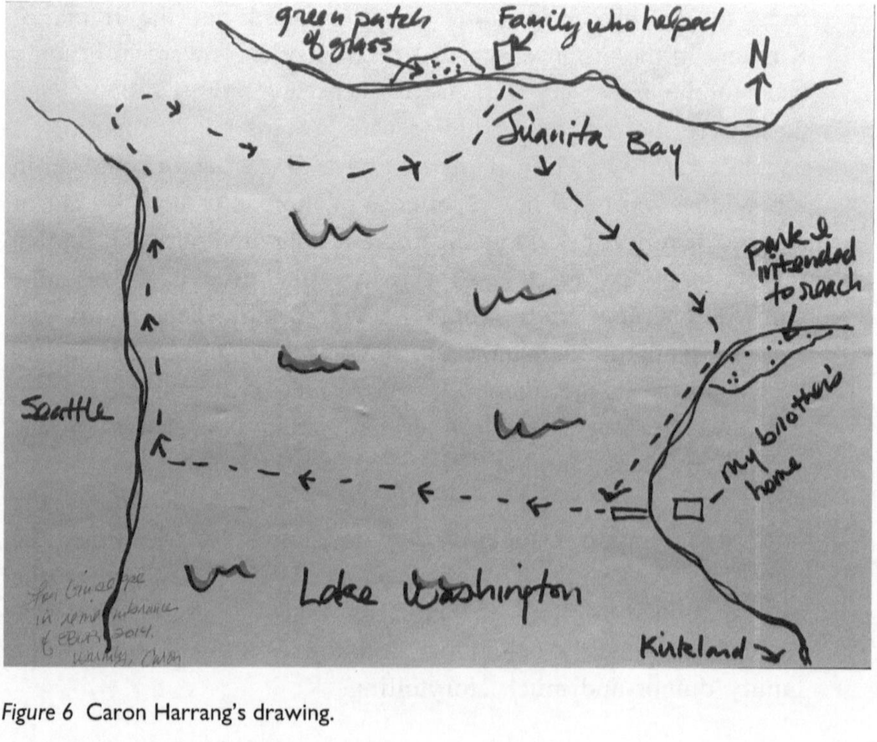

Figure 6 Caron Harrang's drawing.

remark was a withdrawal from that particular atmosphere of intimacy, *like among teenagers*, which we were experiencing. Just to be clear, it is the same atmosphere that found in Antonello Venditti its unparalleled bard.

SELF-NAMING. The analyst who says something private to the patient (*self-disclosure*) in reality performs an act of self-naming, that is, the same act performed by the poet when he places his own name inside the text.[2] It could also be defined as a peculiar form of metalepsis: a character who logically should be part of a different historical and temporal dimension, comes onto the stage – an extradiegetic character, as it is called in narratology. It is the same narrative shortcut of every transference interpretation. Using these two rhetorical techniques, like the poet whose vocative is self-directed, so the analyst comes back time and time again to place himself in the text of the patient's discourse as if he were another subject or a subject *other*; as if he did not only play the roles, as the case may be, of a listener or storyteller, but also of a character.

Self-naming is a general principle of understanding followed in all psychoanalysis models. This is what is meant by the movement summarized in Nerval's 'Je suis un Autre' or in Rimbaud's 'Je est l'autre', one turns to oneself as if it were someone else; and when he turns to others it is as if he were treating them as himself. The amazing duplication of personality reveals the constitutive alienation that lies at the bottom of subjectivity, the theme Lacan has insisted upon so much. Why, then, is self-disclosure so scandalous? Because it insists upon the presumption that the person who speaks on their own behalf knows what they are referring to, that they are, more or less, the master in their own home. As in transference interpretation, so in self-revelation, in a way that is not at all obvious – so much so as to represent for some only a break in the setting – what is uncovered is the unconscious.

There is, then, a second aspect of the self-disclosure or self-naming. It can be seen as a sophisticated rhetorical artifice: as an 'effect of reality',[3] according to the definition given by Roland Barthes. It is the description of small details that seem to be useless in the narrative economy of a novel, but which help to make the reader accept the sacrifice of the naïve realism with which he looks at the things. In this sense, the effect of reality would be oriented not so much towards suspending representation (which is impossible if what is meant by this is the play performed on the scene of the unconscious), but rather, towards armoring the voluntary suspension of disbelief which gives access to the universes of fiction.

SENSIBLE IDEAS. Only 'sensible ideas'[4] should be expressed to the patient, i.e. ideas that cannot be separated from their emotional connotations.

SEXUALITY. It is inherently subversive because, well before social order, it threatens the balanced subject–object distance on which symbolization is based at its zero degree.

SHAME. The most humane of primary emotions since it is based on sociality. Surprisingly, in *Inside Out*,[5] the 3D computer-animated comedy-drama that features as main characters five basic emotions, it is not portrayed. However, one of my patients suggested to identify it in the movie in the *disgust* for oneself as the reflection of that of others. Was it to spare the young audience of animated films the consciousness of the extreme cruelty of which humans turn out to be capable when they deny their neighbour the right to exist?

The fact that shame could become a boulder was portrayed in Figure 7, a drawing by L., an 11-year-old girl.

SIMULTANEITY. For Ogden,[7] the unconscious speaks with a genuineness of which the conscious experience is devoid. Conscious experience helps us to manage practical life, the unconscious to nourish the feeling of existence. When we see things from the point of view of the unconscious, we feel more real and true, because we no longer have just one outlook but many outlooks. Like poetry, the unconscious offers us many simultaneous perspectives on things. But why is it so? If we think of the unconscious as a matter of language, such plurality of perspectives means expanding the individual roots that sink into the fertile soil of sociality

SCEPTICISM. Barthes[8] takes up and appropriates the definition given by one of the followers of Pyrrho of sweetness as the 'final word of scepticism'. A sweet scepticism is a figure of hospitality. On the one hand, following a principle of gentleness, it helps the subject to avoid with elegance and discretion any form of reduction by the other to his own schemes and explanatory principles, even if they are innocent and well-intentioned. On the other hand, it repudiates any form of dogmatism.

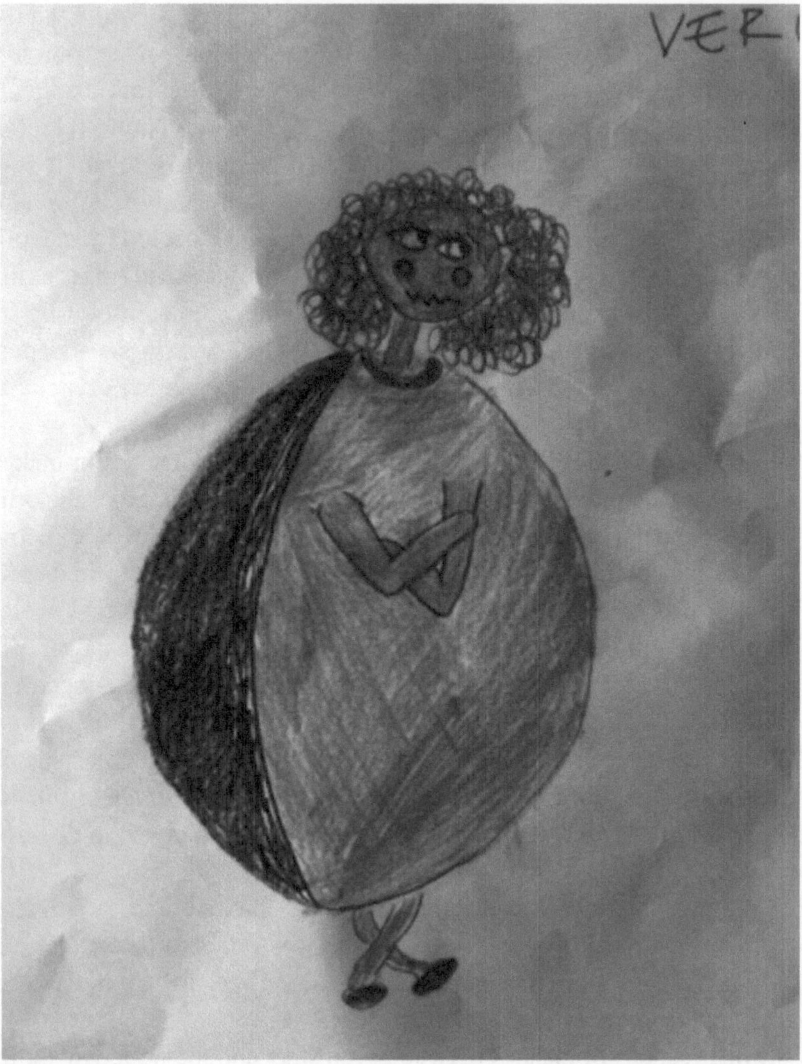

Figure 7 Shame[6]

THE SKY IN A ROOM. Patients who use psychotic defences are like the characters in *Gravity*[9] who are dispersed in outer space. The container object has become infinite and although present, it cannot fulfil its functions of receiving and transforming anxiety.

Sometimes this grows out of measure in the form of expressions of hatred and resentment that threaten to imprison the analyst and the patient in a very sad situation. The only way out is to listen to them as legitimate and desperate attempts to get in touch with the object *in the here and now.* Their relentless repetition would then no longer be the sign of a nucleus of radioactive pain which is difficult to modify, but of precise technical deficiencies of the analyst and of an occluded receptivity. Seen as such, the psychic elements projected at inaccessible distances of space and time are attracted immediately by the centripetal force of the analytic field. The sky is, so to speak, brought into the analytic room and the container reacquires human dimensions and functions.

SKYPE I. Seeing patients on Skype turns us into involuntary filmmakers. We begin to look at our own image along with the image of the other. Every patient (and every analyst) has their own style of directing. Choice of sound effects, background, lighting, frame (whether it's fixed or continuously moving). In short, we are forced to take a crash course in semiotics of the image on video. Nothing is ever pure mechanical recording. Editing work becomes an intrinsic part of analysis.

SKYPE II. Sometimes unexpected events produce special effects. I felt transported to the dreamlike atmosphere of the *One Thousand and One Nights* tale when one day I heard the voice of a muezzin calling to prayer.

In Italy it is Christmas, but not in the country where V. lives. I receive a worried message because she was not able to contact me.

During a session the background noise (because of the internet connection) sounds like the crash of waves.

I hear echoes of clashes between protesters and the police in another country, which one could read about in the newspapers at theat time.

The face of my interlocutor is fixed in a distorted picture which immediately reminds me of the portraits by Francis Bacon. It thus reveals a possible depth of otherwise invisible anguish.

Every four to five minutes the connection is interrupted. A mimesis of other former hypothetical disconnections in the primary relationship with the object.

She puts herself at the bottom corner of the screen. I only see a tuft of hair: 'Snoopy behind his kennel', I think.

SKYPE III. One time the Skype connection crashes so we FaceTime instead or meet on WhatsApp; another time we switch to Viber … caught up in the web!

SKYPE IV. The lack of the intimacy you have when you are physically in the same room is an inherent limitation. All that remains of the sensory shell of the setting – which for Winnicott is nothing less than the maternal womb – is a pale virtual copy.

SPHINX. We've gone from the psychoanalysis of Oedipus, which gives answers to the psychoanalysis of the Sphinx, which simply asks questions.

SPIRAL. Every analytic couple could start off by repeating Nietzsche's oath:

> But we who are different, who are thirsty for reason, want to look as carefully into our experiences as in the case of a scientific experiment, hour by hour, day by day! We ourselves want to be our own experiments, and our own subjects of experiment.[10]

However, it is preferable to set aside the idea of finding a scientific meta-language to secure the truths of the analytic relationship and rather conceptualize the analytic conversation as a virtually infinite spiral movement. The dialogic quality that characterizes it does not 'close', it does not conclude. It is endless and inexorably recursive. The new word interferes (*interferisce*; in Italian the word 'ferisce' means: it wounds) with the old; it influences it, infects it, then retroacts on it. This happens either on the horizontal plane of meaning and the play of signifiers (the 'secular forms [of the unconscious]: the implicit, the indifferent, the additional, the deferred'[11]), or on the vertical level between the various stratifications of the conscious–unconscious discourse that come alive in analytical listening.

STALKER. One wonders whether those who behave like stalkers – in a strict and figurative sense – commit themselves not so much to annoying the victim as to desperately searching for the object. Similarly with serial killers. One might say that it is as if they had delegated to the detectives the reconstruction of their precarious identity profile, by literally succeeding in seeing and recognizing them.

STYLE. That psychoanalysis lies between science and literature is seen from the fact that all great authors create a new world. That's why it will never be possible to get rid of them permanently. Not only because of the need for a historical perspective of the development of the concepts, or of external and internal intertextuality, but because we would renounce the more a-specific, artistic or aesthetic aspects of their understanding of psychic and relational life. There would be no reason to do so. (In addition, a personal note: Winnicott is perhaps the only author who I cannot wait to go back to in the evening after I overcome my laziness and reread one of his books, as I do with my most beloved novels.)

SUBJECT. In the letter known as 'of the seer', Rimbaud – Lacanian ahead of his time – affirms that the Ego is in fact the other.[12] Paradoxically, it could be argued that the animal is indeed a subject, as many by this term understand an entity separate and concluded in itself, because it really lives in itself and is determined solely by the stimuli it receives and by the instinctual responses that they trigger. On the other hand, the human being lives in the Other and never really in himself.[13] Psychoanalysis has built its edifice on the systematic deconstruction of the illusion of the subject. Not everyone, however, realizes this, and, without knowing it, they refer to a pre-Freudian idea of the subject. Only, as they imagine it … with the unconscious encapsulated inside as a perverse homunculus.

SUBLIMATION. While it summarizes Freud's art theory and has passed into everyday language, the concept of sublimation is outdated. Moreover, a certain inconsistency has marked it since its birth. Does it employ sexualized or de-sexualized drive energy? Is it a defence or an alternative to defence? Does it involve Eros or Thanatos? Is it useful or useless in clinical work? Is it about ordinary or exceptional creativity? Is it overly infiltrated by ideology or not? Is it singular or plural? The only handhold, however uncertain, for a definition lies on an extrinsic and 'sociological' criterion of the concrete artistic realization. However, one can try to 'reinvent' it in the light of some principles of the pre-Romantic aesthetics of the sublime. Indeed, both are theories of spiritual elevation, that is, towards abstract thought and of the 'moral' conquests of man, and both try to explain the mystery of the aesthetic experience. On the one hand, the aesthetics of the sublime gives us a modern myth to articulate a series of factors indicated occasionally by various authors as constituents of sublimation, but not inserted in a single and coherent framework: loss and the early work of mourning, the recurrence of a catastrophic factor, the coincidence with a process of psychosomatic categorization that coincides with subjectivation. On the other hand, it allows us to grasp empathically, by living it *from within*, the experience of pleasure more or less unnoticed but intrinsic to any sublimation, and in respect of which it can be proposed as a model.

SUBLIME. To compose his work, Bion used multiple matrices: psychoanalytic, philosophical, mathematical, literary. Out of all of this, the last one is the least explored. True, we know that he mentions many authors of the Romantic period, such as Coleridge, Keats, Blake and Wordsworth, or authors who were exalted in the Romantic period, like Milton. However, the influence on Bion of the aesthetics of the sublime, which is chronologically pre-Romantic, is not as well known, although it marks the Romantic period most fully. Bringing a number of Bion's concepts to this secret symbolic matrix serves a variety of purposes. Firstly, it contributes to the study of sources. Secondly, it makes them appear less casual or idiosyncratic than we could believe, since they are the ones that are less immediately understandable but not of lesser weight (negative capability, O, nameless terror, infinite, language of achievement, *at-one-ment*, and so on). Finally, inserting these notions into a matrix, showing how these elements are not just juxtaposed but dynamically interconnected, greatly helps us to grasp their meaning, not only theoretical but also clinical. In fact, it can rightly be argued that the aesthetic matrix is the one to which Bion has gradually subjected all the others which mattered to him.

SUPER-THEY. 'It's not so much Super-Ego … it's SUPER-THEY!!!'

SUPERVISION. You've got 50 people who are expecting to listen to something new. The local star presents a case where there is not a speck of a psychoanalytically oriented listening, according to *any* model. *What should I do?*

SURPRISE. Theodor Reik[14] wrote an essay about surprise which has since become a classic. In analysis it is just as important as in art. Surprise is a pleasant shock which lives in the negative dimension of the uncanny. The familiar is *altered*, something catches us unprepared, an unexpected guest arrives, the unconscious manifests itself, we find ourselves defenceless in the face of the infinite of the world and of language. It is a painful moment of confusion as a sign of a crisis of the subject, but also of the pleasant reconstruction of a split or of an increase in personalization. If tolerable, that is, if it is possible to retrieve a point of equilibrium immediately, it is therefore a negative pleasure. When it surpasses the ability to immediately regain a safety distance, it may be frightening and traumatizing.

The underlying phantasy to any kind of pleasant surprise is an ecstasy taking place in front of the mother's eyes: an *affection* that *gives meaning* (Dante: 'Love, that in noble heart is quickly caught';[15] or Flaubert: 'And they stared into one another's eyes, both pale and their hands trembling';[16] or Freud:[17] 'When he saw the girl on the floor engaged in scrubbing it, and kneeling down, with her buttocks projecting and her back horizontal, he was faced once again with the posture which his mother had assumed in the copulation scene').

SYMBOLIC. Ever since the access to the symbolic, there is never a pure absence or presence of the object for the subject. In the verbal sign, that has now become essential to think of it (*or even just to perceive it*), the concrete object is always either (at least) retained when absent, or (at least) lost when present. The symbolic performs precisely the function of being able to modulate various levels of absence–presence of the object and of generally being able to have an *indirect* grip on the real. It follows that the so-called concrete thought attributed to psychotics is never entirely such, otherwise they would fall into the utmost aphasia, as may only happen in the most extreme stages of psychic fragmentation.

Notes

1 F. Grassadonia and A. Piazza (directors), *Salvo*, Francia, Italia, 2013.
2 V. Magrelli, 2015, *Millennium Poetry*. Bologna: Il Mulino.
3 R. Barthes, 1989 [1984], *The Rustle of Language*. Berkeley and Los Angeles, CA: University of California Press.
4 M. Carbone, 2010 [2004], *An Unprecedented Deformation: Marcel Proust and the Sensible Ideas*. New York: State University of New York Press.

5 P. Docter (director), *Inside Out*, USA, 2015.
6 I thank S. Boffito for allowing me to reproduce it here.
7 T. H. Ogden, 2003, 'What's true and whose idea was it?', *International Journal of Psychoanalysis*, 84:593–606.
8 R. Barthes, 2002, *Le Neutre. Cours au Collège de France (1977–1978)*. Paris: Seuil, p. 66.
9 A. Cuarón (director), *Gravity*, USA, 2013.
10 F. Nietzsche, 2006, *The Gay Science*. New York: Dover Publications, pp. 39–140.
11 R. Barthes and R. Havas, 1977, 'Ascolto', in: *Enciclopedia*, vol. 1. Turin: Einaudi, p. 989. 'Listening', in: R. Barthes, ed., *The Responsibility of Forms, Critical Essays on Music, Art and Representation*. Trans. R. Howard. New York: Hill and Wang, 1985.
12 A. Rimbaud, 2005, *Rimbaud: Complete Works, Selected Letters*. Chicago, IL: Chicago University Press.
13 See the famous example of Jakob Johann von Uexküll's description of mint life, taken up by G. Agamben, 2002, in his book *L'aperto*. Turin: Bollati Boringhieri, pp. 49–51.
14 T. Reik, 1933, 'New ways in psycho-analytic technique', *International Journal of Psychoanalysis*, 14:321–334.
15 D. Alighieri, 1833, *The Inferno of Dante*. London: Longman, p. 47.
16 G. Flaubert, 1898 [1869], *Sentimental Education: A Young's Man History*. London: H. S. Nichols, p. 9.
17 S. Freud, 1918, 'From the history of an infantile neurosis', *The Standard Edition of the Complete Psychological Works of Sigmund Freud*, vol. 12, pp. 1–124, p. 92.

T

TARANTINO. In his film *The Hateful Eight*[1] Quentin Tarantino uses Sergio Leone's slowing down of time not so much for the rhythm of the images as for the dialogue. Paused, inattentive, ironic, it wanders in a metanarrative and citational dimension. It seems a sort of sublime 'talking-as-dreaming'.[2]

TAXI. *I was in Bassano del Grappa* (in fact, I had never been there before, but a week later I was to hold a seminar there) *and I could not find the place where they were expecting me. I was very anxious at the thought of arriving late. I kept looking for a taxi. Some of them approached me but they were always busy. I walked into a street and immediately realized that it seemed very dangerous. Signs of degradation and anti-burglary railings at all doors and windows, as I have seen only in Brazil. At one point I said: 'But in Bassano del Grappa, in such a small place, such a situation is absurd!'* I woke up.

TEA. 'A smell of tea',[3] S. begins in the corridor. I consider a couple of responses, so to speak, *in* the transference. One might be: 'Barred *Løv*!';[4] a second: 'Dior, *Eau sauvage extreme*!' I cautiously choose to remain silent.

TECHNOLOGY AND SPONTANEITY. Summer of 2013, at the Berlin Zoo, in front of the leopard cage: an enigmatic and beautiful animal. This time, I tell myself, the photo must be perfect (see Figure 8). I focus the Nikon, adjust the various parameters and click. Close to me, I can hear someone laughing good-naturedly. Caught up in my need for technical perfection I did not realize that the leopard, obviously bored of waiting, had lazily moved to the adjacent cell. Similarly, in analysis, in understanding the opportunity of an event (καιρός), there is no time to engage in too much reasoning.

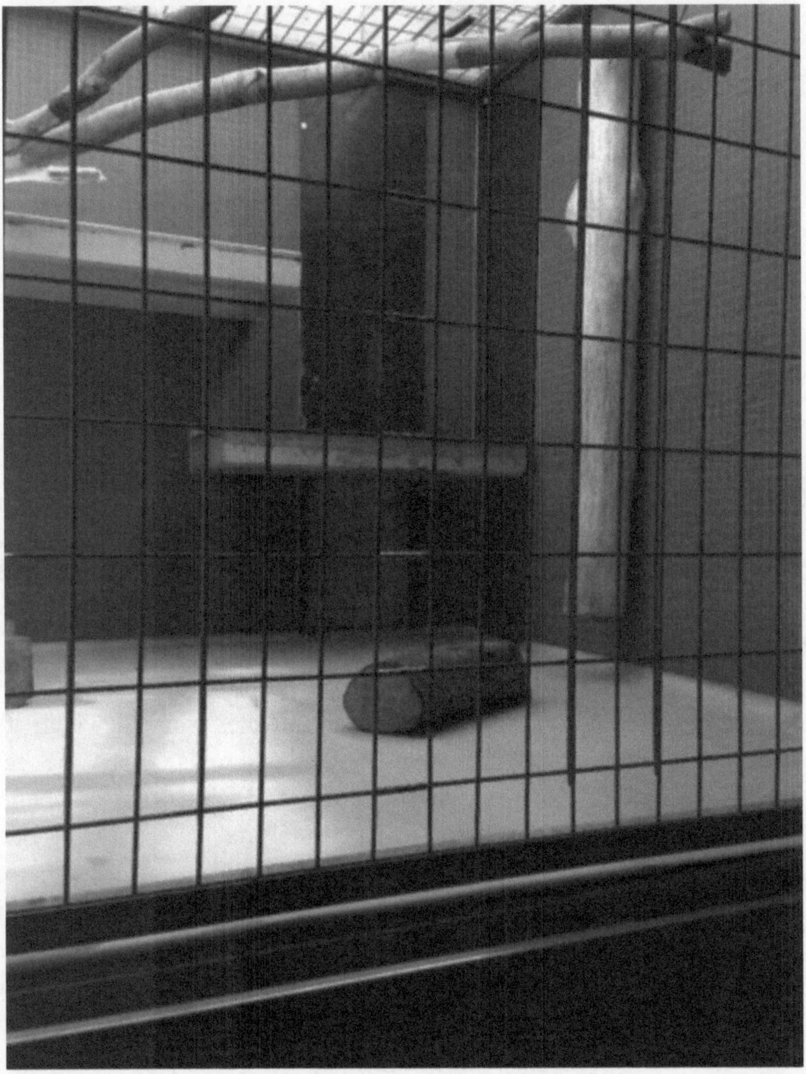

Figure 8 The leopard's cage in the Berlin Zoo

TEMPERATURE. If you have to cook pasta, the water should be boiling. In order for a person to change, the therapeutic relationship should reach the right temperature. Only then will it get to the critical point of the transition state. What are the factors that raise the temperature? Constant increases of L (love), H (hate), K (knowledge). Among the factors that facilitate these increases, an essential one is *time*.

THEATRE WITHIN THEATRE. When at court the group of travelling actors put on the play that Hamlet suggested to them, the tension skyrockets. The narrative mechanism of theatre within theatre has an effect of 'proximization'. A larger narrative dimension is narrowed to a more limited portion, the beginning of a concept. Any work of art fulfils a similar meaning with respect to life. Compared to life and to the fiction *en abîme* of analysis, the dream is but the third level of this infinite game of mirrors. The fascinating phenomenon of a dream within a dream multiplies the reflection up to the point of vertigo. It goes without saying that the advantage of the spectator who is forced to feel like the actor, is that he becomes more fully a subject and therefore a human being.

THOUGHT WITHOUT THE THINKER. Could it be a thought neither guaranteed nor claimed by any authorities of the Ego? A thought in the form of rhythm? Something ineffable in the body as it cannot be represented?

THREAD. In the wooden-reel game of Freud's[5] grandson what we see is that Ernst creates a dramatic, theatrical performance in two acts. He is the playwright and, along with the reel and the string to which it is tied, a character too. The child violently throws away the reel, exclaiming 'a loud, long-drawn-out "o-o-o-o,"' which (not by chance) his mother, who is present at the scene, interprets as a '"*fort*" [gone]' (act I); then, little by little, he pulls it back, exclaiming *da* ('there!') (act II). Freud's interpretation is that the child stands for himself while the reel represents his mother. The role of the string, however, is more mysterious. Interpreted, the story would be: a child and a mother are separated in a violent manner (or rather, a child is abandoned by his mother) and then find each other again. The finale is joyous.

However, in these justly famous pages Freud makes it clear that during the game of 'disappearance and return … *as a rule one only witnessed its first act, which was repeated untiringly as a game in itself*, though there is no doubt that the greater pleasure was attached to the second act'. What is repeated 'untiringly' is above all the 'distressing experience' of the first gesture, which is configured as a true form of 'pleasure of pain', or rather masochism. We are here confronted by another scandal following those just mentioned, concerning people who derive pleasure from beating fantasies or from masochistic behaviour, and who continue always to have the same traumatic dreams. Rooted within the discussion on masochism in 'Beyond the pleasure principle', and introduced by the hypothesis on the significance of traumatic dreams, the wooden-reel game represents its most illuminating model, even if the former is a pathological event and the latter a normative one. Freud could not have intended this in any other way.

So the child seems to feel pleasure in something that in itself is painful: that is, the disappearance of the object.

How might this be explained?

According to Freud, an initial explanation is that the disappearance is *a prelude to rejoicing* at the reappearance. A second explanation is that *active repetition of a suffered event* is preferable to suffering the event passively. A third is that throwing away the reel offers the possibility of *avenging* oneself on a substitute for the frustrating object. In relation to this last, Freud gives us a further indication by hinting at a significant 'instinct for mastery [*Bemächtigungstrieb*] that was acting independently of whether the memory was in itself pleasurable or not', a concept that resonates with that of 'obtaining erotic mastery over an object [which] coincides with that object's destruction'[6] in the oral phase of libidinal organization. Apart from anything else, this association confirms our proposition that the reading of the wooden-reel game should be superimposed on the interpretation of primary pregenital sadism, to which, as we have seen, Freud assigns a key role in the understanding of beating fantasies and the origin of the perversions. Nevertheless, all of this is still insufficient to account for why the child repeats the *first* part of the game above all, as if it were a full game in itself.

But what is Freud saying here? Or rather, what can be intuited from what he is saying?

Let's go back to the game. It is of course customary to emphasize that by throwing away the reel the child controls the disappearance of his mother, with whom from Freud onwards the toy has been identified.[7] What is mostly not seen is that the child does not just throw away 'the mother', but throws *himself* away.[8] Freud has already suggested this idea when a few lines later he describes the boy making himself disappear from the mirror. A double identification would be in play: first with himself as he makes his mother disappear, and second with the reel-as-child that is thrown away.

Whether the reel is identified with the child or with the mother, the first act is (or rather, *appears* to be) always masochistic, because the child procures a form of pleasure by means of pain. This should already make us think that we are dealing with a pleasure different from that of concrete reunion, which he feels when he pulls the reel back with the string and makes it reappear, joyfully exclaiming '*da!*' Indeed, Freud adds,

> the child may, after all, only have been able to repeat his unpleasant experience in play because the repetition carried along with it a yield of *pleasure of another sort* [*ein andersartiger … Lustgewinn*] *but none the less a direct one.*

A pleasure of another sort but none the less a direct one.

But what pleasure?

At this point, Freud surprisingly hints at the 'highly enjoyable' experience (*hoher Genuß*) that can be derived from seeing a tragedy at the theatre (not from suffering it!), and stops there. We know where this will end up: in the death instinct. But could there be an alternative explanation? And what if we could formulate this explanation in such a way as to endorse the first passage on rhythm and the invaluable link back to aesthetic experience that he makes by referring to tragedy (and to art in general)? May we not postulate pleasure of a different kind in the pure repetition of a rhythm? A pleasure linked to the genesis and stabilizing of the Ego rather than to the satisfaction of the impulses of the id? A pleasure that is the fruit of the urge-to-be and that derives from confirmation of the feeling that one exists? But then this repetition would only *appear* to be 'blind'. While being opposed to the pleasure principle according to the traditional notion, it would have nothing to do with the death drive, or else would necessarily entail its redefinition. Significantly, Freud himself hints that a new aesthetic, 'some system of aesthetics with an economic approach to its subject-matter', could lighten these processes. In my opinion, such an aesthetic could focus on the significance of rhythm in the transindividual constitution of the subject.

Contemporary psychoanalysis, centred on the model of psychic birth from the first object relations, gives us the tools for probing deeply into this new aesthetic, but it was Freud himself who tried to do it first. We have the impression that this is exactly what is expressed by the title of our third text, from 1924, 'The economic problem of masochism'. Interestingly, the very title of this text carries a reference to an economy (we could say an 'aesthetic') of the sensations of unpleasure – pleasure at play in masochism. What would this aesthetic consist of? What is the 'tragedy' at which we are present in masochism?

To know more, we must look more closely at the other actor in the *pièce* entitled 'The wooden-reel game': the string. *What does the string stand for?*

Curiously, the Italian word *filarino*, which derives from *filo* (string) and *filare* (to form a sequence, to make sense), means 'the perfect love', and denotes a pair of lovers who have a perfect understanding. *Filare*, however, also stands for *amoreggiare* (to flirt).[9] The string, both in the case of its identification with the mother and in that of self-identification, is the operator that enables recovery of the reel (reel-object in the first case, reel-child in the second). Can we not see this string as the string of memory, as a device that permits us to evoke images of the beloved object, an act that is often prelude to the possibility of finding it again concretely? And would not the first memories we can imagine take the form of ordered rhythms of sensations inscribed in the body?

But then perhaps we would have revealed the secret of the wooden-reel game and the justification for the 'different' pleasure (but now we could say, with greater precision, 'enjoyment') that the child experiences in throwing away his toys. The object *seems* to disappear (and concretely it does: here the wooden reel *stands for* the word – that is, for the psychic representation of the object) but never does so entirely, because *contact is maintained with the string!* The pleasure of the representation (sublimated, or rather transformed into something that allows sight of the 'other') takes the place of the pain of the direct/non-mediated contact with the object that has previously behaved as a frustrating object, and functions as a 'preliminary pleasure' in relation to that experienced at the moment of actual reunion. We see here at work the basic function of emotions of *linking* (in Italian, *legare*) objects together that according to Bion (1959) are at the very foundation of thinking.

But in fact you don't even need to get to the full game to understand what happens, because the first thread (which is not a real thread) is the name/interpretation that Sophie gives to the sound emitted by the child (the *o-o-o-o*). The lost object, which is not yet the spool but another toy thrown under the bed, is magically and simultaneously retrieved in the name (in the symbol) thanks – we would say with Bion – to the maternal capacity for reverie.

So what does the child gain from the play?

Some control over the object, a degree of distance, a certain security, a deferral of trauma. The annihilating terror of dread is transformed into a tolerable and protective anxiety. Throwing a toy and getting it back is of course not the same thing as suffering abandonment by one's mother. Beyond Freud's vignette there is a further factor relating to pure play, because, by impoverishing itself of some qualities, ludic action – Freud calls the perverse action 'a carrying out of the [corresponding] fantasies in play'[10] – it is abstracted/transformed into language (*fort/da*). The word now *stands* first of all for the ludic gesture, which it still accompanies, and then for the Other *tout court*. As Moravia[11] writes, evil is dreadful but the representation of evil is redemptive. *Where it seemed that the child was throwing away the mother (and/or himself), he was in fact only restraining it (restraining himself) in the symbolic representation.* In the game – and by now we are no longer on the concrete plane but a symbolic one – there *is* separation, because it has been enacted, and there is *not* separation: or rather its effects are largely mitigated precisely because the child and his mother remain linked by the string.

As Chemama and Vandermersch[12] astutely write, at a very basic level it is the 'bond of opposition between two syllables of the language with the repetition of the loss and reappearance of the desired object, pleasure and pain, [that] which can define enjoyment' (p. 143).

It is clear that the sublimative transformation from which the subject is born requires a certain psychic work, a suffering that we could already define as *suffering* pleasure. If we leverage on the lexical assonance with the term 'bond' (*legame*), we can also guess what nature can be the process described by Freud of 'tying' (*legare*) the mass of stimuli that in trauma burst into the psyche.

But then can we not see in this game of syllables a pure rhythm expressed in a kind of song? And rhythm itself as the first vehicle of a musical or semiotic meaning, so to speak, which precedes the semantic meaning of the word? In the interpretation that little Ernst's mother, Sophie, gives of what begins as a simple game of syllables, we see this transformation which is always on the point of completion, but also of being undone, and the inevitably transindividual or intersubjective dimension (the *string*, the *bond*, the *linking*) that is the only one in which it can happen. If we did not take account of the role of the other's presence and of language even in its purely rhythmic component, we would not understand how representational concepts are formed, or how the ability to think is developed.

Despite Lacan's insistence on the unconscious as a discourse of the Other, in his discussion of the episode of the *fort/da* game, the role of Sophie (of the maternal presence) as the agent that actually helps turn a signifier into a linguistic sign is not explicitly emphasized. In fact, the *fort/da* game is one composed of two distinct parts: the *fort* and the *da*. In each of these, the first stage consists in throwing the wooden reel and the second (in reality simultaneous) in holding on to it by its name *thanks to the* mother's *interpretation*. The child can make his mother, identified with the wooden reel, 'disappear' and 'reappear' only because she is discreetly present in the room. What is more, her gaze is seconded by that of Freud, who is present at the scene and so can act as the guarantor of a wider consensuality, a thirdness in relation to the accuracy of the mother's interpretation. The scene recounted by Freud is therefore a masterly example of a mother –

and of a father, represented in this case by Freud – who knows how to keep a good distance between herself and her child.

In reflecting on masochism, Freud comes close to rounding off this area of study, though in my opinion the Lacanian reading and the intersubjectivist, post-Bionian psychoanalytic perspective are still necessary for its full theorization. But then, even when Freud sees dreaming as a 'binding' of the stimuli that erupt into the psyche in order to master them, he cannot help but consider dreaming 'social' and, in spite of appearances, never purely individual. Moreover, it is obvious how the first 'masochistic' stage of loss intervenes: only something from which one has been temporarily separated can be bound in the mnemic traces. We can clearly see that the sublimating transformation that gives birth to the subject requires some psychic work, a suffering that we could actually call a *suffering of pleasure*. If we exploit the lexical assonance with the word 'bond' [*legame* in Italian], we can also intuit the possible nature of the process Freud described as 'binding' [*legare*] the mass of stimuli that erupt into the psyche in trauma.

In normal development, in play, and in symbolic representation in general, the child evokes the sense-making/flirting of which this very capability is the fruit, and does so before there is any specific representation of reunion with the object. It is like saying that any happy representation stands by its very nature for a perfect sense-making with the object. Since at birth the infant enters a state of impotence, at its origin primary symbolization cannot help coinciding with symbolization provided by the mother's love, a love that expresses itself in her concrete presence and in her capacity for mental presence, or rather for *reverie* (the first string). Gradually assimilated by the child, this function becomes his own capacity for symbolizing/representing (the second string). With the development of more highly evolved psychic functions, this level of representation will enable self-consciousness and hence responsibility and guilt.

If the subject identifies with the object that maltreats him, he can hope to arouse guilt in it and then a reparative impulse of love. If in turn he attacks the object, he will fall prey to guilt in the same way and will strengthen himself in his positive feeling of reparation towards it. When in relation to the wooden-reel game we emphasize the aspect of control exercised by the subject over the object, we sometimes neglect the fact that there would not be much point to this control outside a link of dependency and love. At the same time, Freud emphasizes that the masochist – considering now 'non-normal' development – only accepts being ill-treated by the love object.

In one of his seemingly simple but astonishing sentences for form and content Winnicott[13] claims that 'In normal growth there is a long period in which the child needs to distinguish between ME and NON-ME aspects of the thumb. The child grasps his thumb and also loves separation from it'. The phrase made me immediately think of the game of *fort/da* because it resonates with Freud's wonder in observing the joy repeated several times both in the launch and in the recovery of the reel. But if the thread indicates that there is in fact no real separation in place, then can it be that the separation of the baby from the spool which we witness as a symbol of the object is only apparent? Wouldn't this point of view introduce gradation in levels of separation rather than a dry presence/absence opposition? One can be present or absent in different ways. Is the material aspect of the thread or word really separate or is it in continuity with the body of the child or of the subject who has fully developed their symbolic ability?

TOY BOX. She asked me if I could keep a box on the shelf, discreet in size but in plain sight, where she would put something at the beginning of every session. And so, she did:

a grain of sand
a one euro cent coin
a grain of Himalayas salt
a yellow Post-it-shaped like a comic bubble
a wax crayon
the word 'control'

Then nothing more …

TRANSFERENCE. Perhaps the therapeutic value of transference interpretation lies not so much in the elucidation of unconscious dynamics as in the increase of temperature and closeness that generates in the relationship an effect of immediacy. The same effect is produced by dreams for their propensity to transference (Freud) and the theoretical-technical concept of the 'dream of the session'. The object attracts the subject and rescues it from the sidereal space in which it was dispersed. It's like the gravitational sling operation with Earth which in *The Martian* by Ridley Scott[14] allows NASA to bring home Mark Watney, the astronaut abandoned by Ares 3 who miraculously survived on Mars.

TRANSFORMATION. The term 'transformation', more than the concept, is very fashionable. Used as a synonym for change it has little or nothing to do with the reasons why Bion makes it the key to his thought. Whether it is intended as an element of the theory of psychoanalytic observation or of a new psychoanalytic theory *tout court*, for Bion 'transformation' is linked to a model of psychoanalysis where the unconscious proto-emotional experience lived in the present of the session is relevant and intended as something that does not belong to either the patient or the analyst, but which is the expression of something *between* the two, of the unconscious intermediate area that is formed in the encounter of two minds. What interests Bion from this point of view is how the 'something between' transforms with respect to the Grid: on the horizontal axis, how it is *used* (not what a certain content means in itself):

> Thus, [he writes] if the content is oedipal material I do not concern myself with this but with the transformation it has undergone, the stage of growth it reveals, and the use to which its communication is being put. This exclusion of content is artificial[…].[15]

In other words, each time a given content is placed in a grid box to deduce the direction of the psychic: whether aiding development or hindering it; whether it leads towards effective concepts and action or the opposite.

TRANSFORMATION IN HALLUCINOSIS. It describes the shift from the hallucination that one had to the ability to recognize it as such. You make the same movement when you wake up from a dream. Like those of night dreams, we can also question the hallucinations we have when we dream while awake.

Here is an example of a micro-transformation in hallucinosis derived from an error in reading the text from a session. A patient,

E., is speaking and she says that she does not know what to expect from analysis, that she is bored, that there are limits but the limits frighten and discourage her. Then the text goes back to the beginning and starts with a capital 'A' with no dot after it. Reading it, I automatically presume that A stands for the analyst and what follows is his response. The text says that she feels frozen, too much under the influence of his family, and in reality, is not entirely present in the consulting room. She says that she suffers because she is not able to rely on others and that all of them only ever speak about themselves. *I realize after a few seconds that it is E. who is still talking!* However, if we refer the text to the analyst, it leads us to think about the possibility that the analyst does not feel valued by the patient, that she suffers from the thought of how her colleagues will judge her work, and that she feels an impulse to give too many clever explanations instead of welcoming E.'s emotions; and finally, that she finds few stimuli in her work. This little blunder could be very useful to understand why the patient insists on complaining that things do not go well with her husband (her 'partner' in analysis?), and that she feels empty and always dissatisfied.

TRANSITIONAL. What is 'transitional' in the *transitional object*? The fact that a single object, material or immaterial, brings together, as does a *concept* at its zero degree, two different and separate terms: in this case, mother and child. The transitional object is a modal operator of the same type as the symbol, the metaphor, or the concept. It builds bridges or connects worlds. The fact that it is material reminds us of the concrete side of any word and the fact that the first concept can only consist of an emotion that connects mother and child, the *at-one-ment* according to Bion. Only thereafter does this 'first concept' become the recognition of an object that, seen with the mother's and the child's eyes, have a 'common', transitional, meaning, and finally, at a more sophisticated level, an abstract meaning. Just like the transitional object can be used *in place* of the mother, so any concept can be used in place of the set of things it refers to. Winnicott mentions the possibility that a transitional object may deteriorate if the relationship with the mother deteriorates. Among the various examples he lists is 'knocking one's head against the wall', a well-known behaviour in very deprived small children. It is not easy to understand how this symptom can represent a transitional object even if it is 'deteriorated'. If it is a transitional object, although deteriorated, it means that it must still represent something that binds the multiplicity of the mother and child into a *unicum*. It may be the *physical pain* of knocking one's head against the wall. Such a case could be a model for masochistic suffering, for a desperate form of pleasure in pain, the equivalent of a fantasy of beating or perversion; all situations where, to paraphrase Freud,[16] one might say that the subject is experiencing a very high enjoyment in witnessing his *own* tragedy.

TRANSLATION. Re-reading a text translated in Google with a few sentences in English, I realize that the programme translated into English some words which also mean something (different) in Italian. So *more* (in Italian 'più') became *blackberries* (in Italian 'more'). It's a kind of mechanical hallucination. Much like our hallucinations or hallucinosis, which are based on the (erroneous) projection of something known onto something which is not. So, for example the English word *due* (in Italian 'l'ammontare dovuto') becomes *two* (the Italian for *two* is 'due').

TRUE SELF. In a brief definitional note Winnicott compares it to an 'Observing Ego',[17] to someone who is present but excluded from the action (or perhaps we should say from *agency*). The association with the idea of the 'normal person hidden, who, like a detached spectator, watched the hubbub of illness go past him'[18] who, according to Freud, is conserved in patients 'in some corner of their mind' and who witnessed the spectacle of psychosis, is obvious. We can also think of delusion as one of the most extreme forms of expression that the false self assumes to defend the 'Observing Ego'/true self. The price you pay for the defensive operation is, as usual, a sense of unreality.

We usually idealize the true self as a fragile and precious part which is forced to hide. In this way, however, we do not see its other side, the *monster*, that which the true self is in the eyes of others; but ultimately, for identification, even in our *own* eyes. The true self is like the Beast waiting to find a Bella who would kiss him and turn him into a handsome prince. How? It is not entirely clear, notes

Barthes, when it comes to this fairytale, but he puts forward a surprising hypothesis:

> Beauty obviously does not love the Beast, but at the end, vanquished (unimportant by what; let us say by the *conversations* she has with the Beast), she, too, says the magic word: '*Je vous aime, la Bête*'; and, immediately, through the sumptuous arpeggio of a harp, a new subject appears.[19]

TRUST.[20] In a wonderful and poetical duet created by Pina Bausch, perhaps the most brilliant contemporary choreographer, we see a couple that moves toward the viewer. Two dancers are wrapped up in heart-rending music. She has a deeply sad face. After two or three steps, she inclines her body to one side, and would fall if it were not for the man who rescues her every time by gently restoring her balance. The scene then repeats and repeats. There is no better picture to define how much an analyst does to help a patient.

Another choreographer, equally inspired, whose performances I have been lucky enough to attend is Alonzo King. Never before had I been moved to tears while watching a modern dance show. The dancers of this company (*Lines Ballet*) move with such harmoniously fluent movements that they become one with the environment around them. They cancel the fracture I/other and I/world which makes us say that we perceive things – while about the animals we say that strictly speaking they have no perception. They restore a primal and happy unity of the body with everything else and give the body an expressiveness that seems reserved only to singing.

I liked the show so much that I decided to go back to see it the day after. In fact, the company performed for two evenings. I bought the ticket even though this time the seat was not that great. I sat down, looked around at the public and recognized many faces from last night's show. *Could they have all had the same idea?!* No, that's not what it was. I discovered that it was one single show split over two nights and even, with disappointment, that my old ticket, was valid for the seat I had last night. Thanks to the hallucination, now become a hallucinosis, I realized how much I wanted to express my joy and my gratitude as a last-minute fan with a kind of hyperbole, even at the expense of my wallet and sense of reality.

Notes

1 Q. Tarantino (director), *The Hateful Eight*, USA, 2015.
2 T. H. Ogden, 2007, 'On talking-as-dreaming', *International Journal of Psychoanalysis*, 88:575–589.
3 Play on words: 'tea' in Italian is 'té', but 'te' means 'you'; so 'Profumo di tè' can be read as 'the smell of tea' but it sounds like 'your smell/perfume/scent'.
4 The name of a brand of tea she noticed a pack on the shelf along the corridor of the office.
5 S. Freud, 1920, 'Beyond the pleasure principle', *The Standard Edition of the Complete Psychological Works of Sigmund Freud*, vol. 18, p. 14 *et seq.* (emphasis added).
6 *Ibid.*, p. 54.
7 But see F. Fornari, 1977, 'I processi di simbolizzazione tra mondo interno e mondo esterno', *Rivista di Psicoanalisi*, 23: 44–62; and J. Derrida, 1987 [1980], *The Post Card, from Socrates to Freud and Beyond*, trans. A. Bass. Chicago, IL: University of Chicago Press.
8 For similarities, see the Heideggerian concept of 'thrownness' [*Geworfenheit*].
9 *Dizionario Treccani*, www.treccani.it/vocabolario/filare3/ (Accessed: June 1, 2018).
10 S. Freud, 1924, 'The economic problem of masochism', *The Standard Edition of the Complete Psychological Works of Sigmund Freud*, vol. 19. London: The Hogarth Press, p. 162.
11 See A. Moravia, 1998, 'L'Argent', in: J. Quandt, ed., *Robert Bresson* (Cinémathèque Ontario Monographs), Toronto, pp. 407–408; see also G. Civitarese, 2012, 'L'*Argent* di Robert Bresson: la redenzione dello stile', www.stateofmind.it/2012/07/largent-di-robert-bresson-la-redenzione-dello-stile/ (Accessed: June 1, 2018).
12 R. Chemama and B. Vandermersch, 2004 [1998], *Dizionario di psicoanalisi*. Roma: Gremese, p. 143.
13 D. W. Winnicott, 1989, *Psycho-Analytic Explorations*. Cambridge, MA: Harvard University Press, pp. 435–436.
14 R. Scott (director), *The Martian*, USA, 2015.
15 D. W. Winnicott, 1984, *Through Pediatrics to Psychoanalysis*. London: Karnac Books, p. 35.
16 Freud, 'Beyond the pleasure principle', cit.
17 Winnicott, *Psycho-Analytic Explorations*, cit., p. 43.
18 S. Freud, 1938, *An Outline of Psycho-Analysis. The Standard Edition of the Complete Psychological Works of Sigmund Freud*, vol. 23, pp. 139–208, p. 202.
19 R. Barthes, 2001 [1977], *A Lover's Discourse*. New York: Hill and Wang, p. 153.
20 www.youtube.com/watch?v=CEns6bHa6iU (Accessed: May 26, 2018).

U

UNBEWUSST. The exercise of silence and doubt in analysis makes it a practice of the negative. The unconscious is negativity by definition or, rather, the fruit of a double negativity, *umbewusst* not only with respect to consciousness but also with respect to the subject because – like language, which in fact constitutes it – it is inherently social. It follows that it is not only the ego which is not a master in its own house: neither is the unconscious.

UNCONSCIOUS I. Let's start by saying what the unconscious is *not*. It is not the animal unconscious nor the neurological one. It was not less *invented* than it was discovered. It is not a unified concept: many models of the unconscious are present in Freud's work. Different models of unconscious have been elaborated upon by leading authors such as Klein, Fairbairn, Winnicott and Bion. Whenever we alter even just a few of the principles of metapsychology, it is clear that the whole idea of the unconscious is changed. For analysts the concept of the unconscious is a bit like that of time. Saint Augustine said that if you ask yourself, you seem to know very well what it is. However, if you have to explain it, then you do not know it anymore. The common idea of having a fairly unified and a well-defined concept of it is false. Most analysts work with a concept of the unconscious which, upon closer inspection, would look like a kind of mythological creature or a patchwork. This is only a problem for those who hold a scientific view of psychoanalysis and for those who have the illusion that one can eliminate all differences. It is not a problem for those who think that, given the complexity of the subject matter, the various theoretical perspectives can also be conceived as intuitive or poetic visions of something that can only be approximated, but never really known, in the sense of possessed. In this sense it is as if they themselves were the fruit of the multiplicity of perspectives that the unconscious creates about things and thanks to this they seem true and real. By definition, the unconscious is unknowable. One can only stand waiting for it to appear indirectly. The unconscious, as Bion would say, does not exist at birth, and must be absorbed from the mother. It therefore constitutes a 'psychoanalytic function of the personality' which manifests itself in dreaming-thinking. It is the faculty, which is both spontaneous as for innate preconceptions and acquired because somebody has to pass it on to the infant, that gives a personal meaning to the experience. Now, is it not possible to think of the unconscious as the virtually infinite totality of language that the subject obviously cannot dominate and which – thanks to a thousand unpredictable, conscious or unconscious, and semiotic or semantic, cross-references between words – always makes him say something different from what he meant consciously?

This is Lacan's famous *ça parle*. The naïve concept of the subject as something closed in itself is floored for the second time. Not a reversal of hierarchy within the subject but *between* the subject and the group. The unconscious coincides with all the infinite effects of meaning virtually deposited in language and for which the subject represents only a crossroads, a place of transit, and a resonance of voices that transcend it. In a conception of this kind, repression is conceptualized in a wider framework and dynamics, less related to the vicissitudes of representations, and more describable in terms of the container/content ratio.

It is clear that if the unconscious is no longer thought of as the cauldron where the most demonic impulses prevail, but rather as a writing system or a symbolizing apparatus, from the point of view of therapy, what matters is not translating the unconscious into conscious (if not as a tactical move) but rather rendering unconscious that which at first needs to be thought of consciously. Perhaps this is why in *Cogitations* Bion[1] translates *unbewusst* (unconscious) as 'unconscioused', which allows us to derive the infinitive verbal form 'to unconscious'. Moreover, if language is the common room where we live and are recognized as persons, and at the same time the conceptual framework which we use to interpret reality, all that stands as eccentric compared to the normative values expressed by it can be a source of psychic suffering. That's why we can say that the individual has a drive for truth, that truth is food for the mind, and that a mind deprived of truth (consensuality) loses strength and falls ill.

UNCONSCIOUS II. The unconscious makes no distinction of circumstance. A small error on the analyst's part can be painted in the dreams of the patient with the crudest colours.

UNIO MYSTICA. In mystical literature, Bion seeks words for a lover's discourse that in his work feels more and more central to analysis. Mysticism offers, among other things, the advantage that a priori everything is shifted/elevated/sublimated into a meeting that by definition can never be carnal.

In more everyday terms, a patient of mine defined transference love as 'a ruled-out love' (*amore barrato*), as suggested by the vowel in *Løv*, a tea brand which she spotted on a bookshelf in the corridor.

UNISON I. In Ingmar Bergman's *Cries and Whispers*, after a period of silence, the sisters Karin and Maria are finally able to talk passionately, but the viewer cannot hear what they say. Instead of the words, the director put in a piece of music for cello by Bach. The scene reminds one of the pre-eminent position the musical or aesthetic element hold over the logical-rational element in analysis.

UNISON II. About mother–child tuning moments, the Boston School of Attachment Theory speaks of 'a dyadic expansion of consciousness'. To indicate the specifically human capacity of cooperation that differentiates us from animals, Tomasello[2] instead uses the expression 'cooperative intentionality'. I wonder if one could see the moment of unison/*at-one-ment* more like a process that aims at (and in the meantime expresses) a matching of intentionalities, pursuing a goal which is fore-seen as shared.

Notes

1 W. R. Bion, 1992, *Cogitations*. London: Karnac Books, p. 353.

2 M. Tomasello, 2014, *A Natural History of Human Thinking*. Cambridge, MA: Harvard University Press.

V

VERTEX. Bion makes a hierarchal distinction between a *vertex* and a *model*. The first refers to the emotional attitude on the part of the analyst, whether they are open to the new or dogmatically enclosed in what they already know. The second, less important, refers to the theoretical option declared and used in clinical work.

VERTIGO. Google allows you to verify how many times an expression occurs in the universal language database. Being accompanied by the adjective 'vertiginous' the noun 'neckline' has no rivals. And 'gravid with vertigo', as Dino Campana defines the breasts of the 'the noble matronas of Spain/With their turbid and angelic eyes'[1] in his poem *Journey to Montevideo*. This is just a confirmation of the truth that any dictionary has already made us aware of, that the most common hallucinosis which we experience is the erroneous feeling that space revolves around us, due to the powerful attraction of the breast, the term analysts use to indicate the (partial) object with which the little child relates to at birth. We don't use this adjective in the same way for faces. Is this not the best evidence that the aesthetic conflict, as Meltzer describes it, should be backdated and moved from the visual to the tactile register?

VORTEX. In Edgar Allan Poe's short story 'A descent into the maelström' we read:

> Never shall I forget the sensations of awe, horror, and admiration with which I gazed about me. The boat appeared to be hanging, as if by magic, midway down, upon the interior surface of a funnel vast in circumference, prodigious in depth, and whose perfectly smooth sides might have been mistaken for

> ebony, but for the bewildering rapidity with which they spun around, and for the gleaming and ghastly radiance they shot forth, as the rays of the full moon, from that circular rift amid the clouds which I have already described, streamed in a flood of golden glory along the black walls, and far away down into the inmost recesses of the abyss.[2]

And further on:

> [...] a great change took place in the character of the whirlpool. The slope of the sides of the vast funnel became momently less and less steep. The gyrations of the whirl grew, gradually, less and less violent. By degrees, the froth and the rainbow disappeared, and the bottom of the gulf seemed slowly to uprise. The sky was clear, the winds had gone down, and the full moon was setting radiantly in the west, when I found myself on the surface of the ocean, in full view of the shores of Lofoden, and above the spot where the pool of the Moskoe-ström *had been*.[3]

What Poe describes in this fascinating story is a natural vortex which is obviously an allegory for an emotional vortex. Likewise, using the model of vortices studied in physics, we can imagine the turbulence of the analytic field. There are many impressive representations of this also in painting. For example, William Turner and his *Storm at Sea* (1824),[4] *A Mountain Pass* (1830),[5] or *Snow Storm – Steam-Boat off a Harbour's Mouth* (1842).[6]

But how are vortices formed?

Vortices, we read in the Treccani dictionary, are generated when two currents that proceed at different speeds come into contact, they are created and destroyed, propagated and dispersed, change shape and size, and their duration is more limited the greater the turbulence of the current.[7] Vortices have a roundabout configuration, which suggests that for a period of time you do not know which may be the 'exit' direction. One of their features is complexity, which is why they cannot be described easily.

In analysis, vortices are created by fluids of turbulent emotions, from the encounter and clash of bodily movements and their kinaesthesia between the analyst and the patient. The characters in the field help to 'guess' or to understand its nature. Since the turmoil that interests us is, for the most part, that which belongs to the present, we must transform into characters all entities that appear in the field narratives.

The protagonist in Poe's story is saved because he clings to a barrel that brings him to the surface. For the analyst the barrel is the theories that should allow him, like a Brechtian actor, to estrange himself from the part recited and to 'show it'.

Giorgio Agamben also wrote about vortices, inspired by a note of Benjamin's, which makes it into a figure of origin as immanent to the present. A vortex arises from the clash of a stream of water against an obstacle or between two streams of water flowing in opposite directions. In it, this struggle between forces is composed in a new form characterized by its *rhythm*. The new form attracts the elements that are in close proximity to its movement. The vortex statue, observes Agamben, is singular. It is a form in itself, narrow and well-circumscribed but at the same time confused with the medium to which it belongs. It follows its own laws, but nothing belongs to it. The keyword here is 'rhythm'. What the author is describing is quite comparable to the idea of rhythm as something that affects time and thereby defines the singularity of the subject. The (emotional) 'vortices' of the analytical field (of the therapeutic relationship) are virtually opportunities for the subject for (re)birth.

Finally, in *Signs* Merleau-Ponty uses the image of the vortex to represent 'the whole of the spoken language'[8] around the child, who swallows it up taking it from noise to meaning.

VIENNA. A locally renowned colleague practically prevents me from reading my work, shocked by Bion's rejection of the Freudian opposition between the primary and secondary process. Unfortunately, he makes me lose my temper, and it all ends up in a big mess. Perhaps regretting this, later, he says: 'You know, here in Vienna we are very attached to Freud'.

Notes

1 D. Campana, 1914, *Canti orfici*. Marradi: Tipografia F. Ravagli, p. 40 (my translation). www.letteraturaitaliana.net/pdf/Volume_9/t238.pdf (Accessed: July 8, 2018).

2 E. A. Poe, 1909, *The Selected Tales of Mystery*. London: Sidgwick & Jackson, p. 211.
3 *Ibid*., p. 216.
4 www.tate.org.uk/art/artworks/turner-storm-at-sea-d25373 (Accessed: January 3, 2019).
5 www.tate.org.uk/art/artworks/turner-a-mountain-pass-d25213 (Accessed: June 13, 2016).
6 www.tate.org.uk/art/artworks/turner-snow-storm-steam-boat-off-a-harbours-mouth-n00530 (Accessed: January 3, 2019).
7 www.treccani.it/vocabolario/vortice/ (Accessed: November 11, 2016).
8 M. Merleau-Ponty, 1964, *Signs*. Evanston, IL: Northwestern University Press, p. 40.

W

WINNICOTT I. I do not know whether it is true, but I have been told this anecdote more than once. Apparently, when invited to lecture in America, Winnicott turned up with a gun and threatened to use it if someone dared to say that his was not true psychoanalysis.[1] I am afraid that if Winnicott's threat were to be carried through and the joke should be put into practice, very few colleagues would be saved.

WINNICOTT II. His book *The Child, the Family and the Outside World* can be read as an extraordinary manual of psychoanalytic technique … a manual with a soul.

WORDPLAY. B. starts the session by telling me that she feels like fighting because she is unwell and that with her husband things have gone from 'bad' to 'disastrous'. He is always tired, in the evening he goes to sleep straight away and they no longer have an intimate life. I suggest that maybe they are rather going from 'bed' to 'disastrous'. This could be another instance in which we could use the concept of 'trasnformation in play': to indicate the moments when, as in jokes, the phonetic and semantic fluidity of language are used to activate the unconscious thought and to rediscover language's openness and plasticity. Le Guen[2] points out that:

> playful thought exploits, plays with attention, and makes fun of it […] it is about the skillful finding of similarities between dissimilar things, to quickly link foreign representations to one another, to reconcile the irreconcilable […] a technique similar to that of working with dreams, because it is about creating a network of unexpected connections using the condensation technique.

Logic would be bypassed, cheated, stunned by the fireworks of words of multiple meanings, to the point of 'making the nonsense seem acceptable and sensible'. The goal is of course the 'pleasure shared with another who shows a "psychic agreement"'.

WRITING I. In an interview published in *Fort Da* after the publication of his first novel, *The Parts Left Out*, Thomas H. Ogden[3] says he does not see any particular difference between writing essays of psychoanalysis and writing a work of fiction. I got the impression that I finally grasped the secret of his incredible creativity. From the outset, he must have taken up essay writing with the same rigour regarding language that even a person completely undrawn to writing would have if they wanted to write a story or a novel. The fact is that in psychoanalysis writing is (like) writing literature and not like writing an essay of, say, psychiatry or epidemiology. If we were more aware of this, our style would immediately improve. This is evidenced by the literary quality of some of the most important authors in the history of psychoanalysis: Freud and Winnicott of course, but also, in their own way, Melanie Klein, the inventor of the extraordinary horror genre, and Bion, with his outlandish mathematics like in *Alice in Wonderland*.

WRITING II. There is truth in Derrida's intuitive although paradoxical thesis that writing precedes speaking. In fact the best ideas come not *before* writing but in the process of writing. We do not write to communicate to others what we know about a certain thing, but to learn what we can yet know about it; and, if anything, to ask others to share what they know by responding to our appeal. It is as if the thought was reconnected to the play of signs from which, from a combination of traces, originated, and in that, resumed momentum and vigour. After all, analysts ask their patients to give up the (relative) transparency of the concept (of words) to indulge in a game of signifiers. You find a similar thought in a didactic but wonderful book by Winnicott, *The Child, the Family and the Outside World*:

> Just as a writer is surprised by the wealth of ideas that turn up when he puts his pen to paper, so the mother is constantly surprised by what she finds in the richness of her minute-to-minute contact with her own baby.[4]

Notes

1 In this 'classic way', and just with 'un peu de honte' (*ipse dixit*) I've been adressed by Paul Denis at the 2018 CPLF Congress in Gênes: mine, he said, is 'a noumenic psychoanalysis and a non-psychoanalytic psychology'. I publicly thanked him for giving me such nice example of dogmatism and ideological use of theories and, together, a gracious opportunity to vaccinate once more against it.

2 C. Le Guen, 2008, *Dictionnaire freudien*. Paris: PUF.

3 T. H. Ogden, 2013, 'The parts left out', *Fort Da*, 19:63–82.

4 D. W. Winnicott, 1975, *The Child, the Family and the Outside World*. Harmondsworth: Penguin Books, p. 25.

X, Y and Z

ZIG-ZAG vs. U-TURN. In a session of supervision, U. (the male patient) and N. (the female analyst) duel from beginning to end. He starts by saying that he is thinking of integrating the cure with hypnosis and with a technique of NLP (Neuro-Linguistic Programming). She confronts him and interprets that he is resisting the analysis. U. does not feel understood, N. feels devalued. U. adds that he sometimes leaves the session as if he had been hit by a truck. N. interprets that he is asking her not to 'beat' him anymore. U. answers something like 'Don't be so touchy!' Meanwhile I've been thinking for a while that N. should practice a little more 'hypnosis' with U. She should allow him to sleep so that he might perhaps dream, and that she herself should give herself time and ways to do the same. Suddenly, looking distractedly at the written text of the session, their initials take on new meanings in my eyes, beyond the practical use of noting down the turns of speech. The 'N' of N. seems to me like the trajectory of a zig-zag, and the 'U' of U. like that of a U-turn. I then got an ideographic representation of the emotional state that prevailed in the field, made of chases, escapes, rapid changes of direction to try to lose track, as seen in action or espionage movies. At a certain point U. tells N. that the analysis should have to do with metaphysics, and we can think that he is asking her to go beyond/μετα the surface. Maybe N. should listen to the characters of 'hypnosis' and 'NLP', which U. imagines would help him to quit smoking, as indications to make the air in the analysis room more breathable and try to experience the mutual dependency as less toxic.

Synoptic headings